A FAMILY GUIDE
TO DEATH AND DYING

A FAMILY GUIDE TO DEATH AND DYING

JIM TOWNS

Tyndale House
Publishers, Inc.
Wheaton, Illinois

*Dedicated in memory of a lovely lady who
lived for others and paid the price of my
knowledge concerning grief: my mother,*
MONA HANCOCK TOWNS

All Scripture references are from *The Holy Bible,*
New International Version, copyright 1978 by New
York International Bible Society.

First printing, August 1987

Library of Congress Catalog Card Number 86-51352
ISBN 0-8423-0830-X

CONTENTS

PREFACE

Death is not an elective, but learning about death is! The subject is as old as life. Although television has brought it into our living rooms, we are still shocked when death touches us personally. Being saturated with death through the mass media doesn't prepare us for dealing with it. Perhaps we have been conditioned to believe that death happens only to "other" people. But the truth is that someone we love very dearly has died recently or will one day become terminally ill and die.

Perhaps you don't feel like reading about death and dying right now. If you are facing death, in the recent past or near future, you would best describe your feelings as hurt, shock, or unreality. At the moment, all you may need to do is to read the contents page. Even that much will help you to decide what you need to read in order to find immediate encouragement.

After reading the section you need to understand right now, you may want to put the book aside and come back to it later so that the complete book can help you help yourself on your own pilgrimage through life.

ACKNOWLEDGMENTS

No one ever writes a book alone, no matter what the title page says. It is not possible in syllable or sentence to express my appreciation for the influence and concern of the many people who encouraged me in this work.

I am indebted to many people whose ideas have slipped unconsciously into my life-style, ideas which may have surfaced here as my own. I have tried to give credit where I can, but I can never acknowledge them all.

I am deeply grateful to Dr. Joy Reeves for the opportunity to teach the death and dying course; Dr. Dick Hurzeler for his continued encouragement; Dr. Beverly Robinson for her professional insights; Dr. Heber Taylor for his kindness in permitting me to be academically interdisciplinary; and the other people who have shared their experiences with me at conventions, seminars, and classes. Their life experiences became information for this book.

Special appreciation is expressed to Mahona Pike, who enthusiastically typed the manuscript; Mr. and Mrs. Erle Morgan, the prayer warriors; and Tyndale House Publishers for their assistance in presenting these ideas to you.

INTRODUCTION
THE FACTS OF
LIFE AND DEATH

Every death is a touching love story, a unique and special drama, just as each birth is. Both birth and death are experiences with deep meaning, neither of which we should avoid.

Sex and death, we used to be told, were taboo as topics of conversation. In the 1970s we learned to talk about sex. In the 1980s we are learning to talk about death. Many books about death and dying have flooded the market and probably there will be more. This one, I hope, will make a special contribution to our understanding about death as being a fact of life and something we should accept as surely as we accept the birth of a child.

Our society has very little time to give to illness, dying, and death. These times of life we would like to handle quickly, get them out of the way, and forget them. Yet the grief remains, and in a society that has a pill or prescription for almost everything, very little is being offered on a long-term basis to help the person struggling through the physical-emotional-spiritual hurricane of illness, dying, and death.

Though death is a fact of life, many try to deny it. One

of my friends described death as "an ever-present boundary to life, which causes us to find meaning in life; yet if we constantly dwell upon death, life will never be lived!" The subjects of illness, dying, and death are ignored and denied by most people, as if we think that someday the medical world will completely conquer them. Realistically, we know that it is not going to happen. We are all going to die, either suddenly or through a long, drawn-out, complicated illness of some kind.

The question is not "If something should happen to us." The truth is "When something happens to us," we will die. It is only a matter of time for all of us. This truth does not have to be depressing, since death is as much a part of life and development as being born was. The writer of Ecclesiastes said, "There is a time for everything: . . . a time to be born and a time to die" (3:1, 2).

Any one of us who has seen illness, dying, and grief, directly or indirectly, will remember. If we are dying or either losing or have lost someone, we probably feel suddenly alone in an alien world. Our body feels desperately weary, our emotions raw. We feel as if we have gone through a blender and the physical, mental, emotional, and spiritual pain is real. We are convinced that life itself is being destroyed. We don't know how to think or how to stop feeling, what to do, and what not to do. Knowledge can't erase the many kinds of pain we are feeling, but certain knowledge can help guide us to some insights that will help us as well as others.

Illness, dying, and death should cause us to appreciate life and to live more sensitively and deeply. The Psalmist wrote, "Teach us to number our days aright, that we may gain a heart of wisdom" (90:12). It seems paradoxical, but it is only when we are confronted by death that we gain such wisdom.

Man has always reacted with fear and fascination to

his concerns with death and dying. He has sought answers to his questions through religion, philosophy, and
education. The theologian wants to know what God has
said about life, death, and the afterlife. The biologist is
trying to define death and when it actually occurs. The
psychologist is concerned with how a person faces his
own death as well as the reactions to the deaths of
significant others in the lives of his clients. The sociologist is investigating how value systems, life-styles, and
attitudes of societies cause people to deal with illness,
death, and dying. The philosopher, poet, and artist are
trying to describe the experience of a life here on earth
coming to an end.

Perhaps we have been too cautious in overprotecting
people from thinking about death in a deeply personal
way. Without reservation I hope to reveal in this book
what I regard as some of the most profound and useful
insights I have learned about illness, death, dying, and
grief. We have a better chance of dealing realistically
with death, for us and our loved ones, if we realize in
advance that it could happen to any of us at any time.

The book is divided into three parts. Part One deals
with illness and provides some insights into caring for
the ill. Part Two deals with death and dying and gives
some answers concerning the process of dying. Part
Three deals with grief, describing the normal grief process and how one deals with the loss of a loved one. The
tools offered in this book have been forged in the fires of
experience and have proven to be effective.

I have drawn on several different parts of my background in the preparation of this book. The first is personal experience. In the last few years, I have lost
several family members. Many of my close friends have
died also, so the topic has become very much a part of
my life.

Much of the book is drawn from my own research

and teaching experience. I have been involved in teaching death and dying courses in the Department of Sociology in my university.

My counseling experience has proven another rich source of information for this book. As I speak at seminars, workshops, conferences, and conventions, as well as in counseling, I have gleaned many insights from others' personal and professional experiences that I believe will be helpful to others.

From observation and reflective thinking, from learning how to ask the questions of why and how concerning the things that happen to us, I've gained much. Through intellectual-emotional-spiritual analysis, many insights and answers have come.

I have drawn heavily on my knowledge and understanding of the Scriptures, which give the basic fundamentals concerning life and death. Along the way, I have counted on the illumination of the Holy Spirit, who empowers the believer to know things beyond human understanding.

I hope this book will provide some new insights and comfort, and motivate you to help yourself.

PART I
ILLNESS

ONE
BILL OF RIGHTS
FOR PATIENTS
AND RELATIVES

There is rarely a need to get involved with hospitals or health-care professionals when we are enjoying good health. But when illness comes or when we have to seek medical attention for ourselves or someone we love, the world becomes strange and often frightening.

In 1972, the American Hospital Association developed and adopted a document entitled "A Patient's Bill of Rights." Although this document is not legally binding in all states, most hospitals use it to provide guidelines for patient care. Some health professionals are apprehensive, because more and more they are fearful of malpractice lawsuits. As the professionals understand their obligations and responsibilities to the patients, they are better prepared to give competent care and seldom need to worry about being taken to court.

As the general public seeking health care becomes better informed about their rights, they take a more active role in the procedure, resulting in the medical professionals listening more effectively to patients and their needs.

PATIENT'S BILL OF RIGHTS[1]

The American Hospital Association developed this document with the expectation that it would contribute to more meaningful and effective medical care. The relationships of the patient, his family, his physician, nurses, and hospital organization take on a new dimension when the process of health care follows these guidelines.

1. *The patient has the right to considerate and respectful care.* According to this right, the patient is entitled to courteous behavior during the time he is under care of health professionals. The personalities of hospital administrators, doctors, and nurses differ. Yet, as a patient, one has a right to expect to be treated as a person of value, dignity, and respect.

2. *The patient has the right to obtain from his physician complete current information concerning his diagnosis, treatment, and prognosis.* This information should be given in terms that the patient can understand.

When it is not medically advisable to give such information to the patient, the information should be made available on his behalf to an appropriate person. The patient, or this responsible person, has the right to know, by name, the physician responsible for coordinating the patient's health care.

The patient has the right to understand his diagnosis, treatment, and prognosis. Since doctors are usually in such a hurry, not all of them take the time to communicate with their patients. The patient worries if he or she has not been given a complete explanation. If the situation permits, the patient should ask questions of the doctor before going into the hospital. The patient should seek some understanding of the medical terminology used by the professionals.

3. *The patient has the right to receive from his physician information necessary to give informed consent prior to the start of any procedure or treatment.* Except

in emergencies, such information for informed consent should include, but not necessarily be limited to, any specific procedure or treatment, the risks involved, and the probable duration of incapacitation. Where there are alternatives for care or treatment, or when the patient requests information concerning medical alternatives, the patient has the right to know about them. The patient also has the right to know the name of the person responsible for the procedure or treatment.

"Consent" is a free, rational decision that presupposes that the patient, or the one responsible for him, has knowledge about that for which consent is given. In order to give informed consent to agree to certain procedures, the patient must have a thorough comprehension of what is involved in the procedures and their consequences, and alternative treatments available. The patient should know the positives and negatives concerning the expected benefits. If he does not understand, he should question the medications and therapies being given. There was a time when the general public thought they were at the mercy of the health professionals and could not ask questions. The physician does have the responsibility to give the patient information.

4. *The patient has the right to refuse treatment to the extent permitted by law, and to be informed of the medical consequences of his action.* The patient can change his mind and refuse a treatment or procedure that he is not fully convinced is necessary. Although he may refuse any treatment, he may be asked by the administrators to sign a form which releases the hospital from any liability for the consequences of his refusal.

5. *The patient has the right to every consideration of his privacy concerning his own medical care.* Case discussion, consultation, examination, and treatment are confidential and should be conducted discreetly. Those not directly involved in the case must have permission from the patient to be present.

21

The patient has the right to be examined by only those professionals who are essential to his care or therapy. Any other observers on the staff must obtain permission from the patient, who may or may not be interested in participating in education or research programs by permitting others to observe his treatment. In the event of death, the rights of privacy are delegated to the surviving relatives.

6. *The patient has the right to expect that all communications and records pertaining to his care should be treated as confidential.* The patient has the right to know how the information will be handled and how much will be related to others. Physician-patient relationships are usually kept confidential, and if there is any question, the patient should discuss his feelings about confidentiality to avoid any instance of miscommunication.

7. *The patient has the right to expect that a hospital must make reasonable response to the request of a patient for services.* The hospital must provide evaluation, service, and referral as indicated by the urgency of the case. When medically permissible, a patient may be transferred to another facility only after he receives complete information and explanation concerning the needs for the alternatives to such a transfer. The institution to which the patient is to be transferred must first have accepted the patient for transfer.

If a hospital does not have adequate facilities or equipment to serve the patient's health need, the hospital should make arrangements for the patient to be transferred to another facility that can provide better treatment and care.

8. *The patient has the right to obtain information as to any relationship of his hospital to any other health-care and educational institutions insofar as his care is concerned.* The patient has the right to obtain information as to the existence of any professional relationships among individuals, by name, who are treating him.

This means that the patient has the right to know about the relationship of his doctor and the hospital with educational institutions such as universities, medical schools, convalescent centers, and private care.

9. *The patient has the right to be advised if the hospital proposes to engage in or perform human experimentation affecting his care or treatment.* The patient has the right to refuse to participate in such research projects.

Hospitals in which research is being conducted are required to take specific measures to protect the patients. A committee must determine whether the research is sound and if the benefits outweigh the risks. If a patient participates in experimental research, he has the right to withdraw from the program at any time he desires. If he suspects that he is involved in experimentation for which he has not given consent, the patient should question his physician and let his wishes be known.

10. *The patient has the right to expect reasonable continuity of care.* He has the right to know in advance what appointment times and physicians are available and where. The patient has the right to expect that the hospital will provide a mechanism whereby he is informed by his physician or a delegate of the physician of the patient's continuing health-care requirements following discharge.

When the patient is discharged from the hospital, he has the right to know when and where his next appointment and treatment will be. He should also be instructed as to his taking care of himself away from the hospital. Since health records are an extremely important factor in one's continuing health care, the patient has the right to keep his records. If he should move, he would need a complete record of his previous treatments. Although the piece of paper belongs to the doctor and hospital, the information belongs to the patient, so he is entitled at least to copies of his records.

11. *The patient has the right to examine and receive an explanation of his bill regardless of source of payment.* Hospital administrators have the responsibility to provide patients with a detailed documentation of costs of services and supplies. Patients are entitled to a complete explanation of the bill and each aspect of it. Patients should ask questions until they know what all the charges mean.

12. *The patient has the right to know what hospital rules and regulations apply to his conduct as a patient.* The patient has the right to have explained to his satisfaction all rules, regulations, and policies of the hospital that are of concern to him. The hospital usually provides a pamphlet that explains this information and the regulations about a stay in the hospital.

THE FAMILY'S RIGHTS

In addition to the patient's rights, there are also rights for the relatives of the patient. Make Today Count is an organization that counsels terminally ill patients, their families, friends, and physicians. This organization has presented a "bill of rights"[2] for the relatives. These self-explanatory rights are meaningful to the family as well as to the patient. The following is a list of the relatives' rights along with suggestions concerning the patients, the relatives, and the hospitals and doctors concerned.

1. *From the very beginning, open and honest communication among all family members is essential.* In cases of terminal illness, the fact of the illness and the possibility of death at an earlier age than otherwise expected must be faced and discussed without reservation. Such knowledge makes it easier for everyone to adjust.

2. *Spouses have the right to learn about the family financial matters.* With such knowledge, they will be prepared to carry on in the event of the incapacitation or absence of the terminally ill patient.

3. *Relatives have a right to peace of mind concerning the patient's affairs.* The relatives of the terminally ill patient will find it easier to carry on in case of the death of the patient if the patient's affairs are put in order, the will made out, and the funeral preferences expressed.

4. *The relative of the terminally ill patient has the right and obligation to take care of his own needs.* Even though he may be accused of being selfish, he must do what he has to do to keep his own peace of mind so that he can better meet the needs of the patient. Each person will have different needs, such as a night out, the opportunity to watch a favorite television program, or perhaps a walk on the beach. These needs must be satisfied. The patient will benefit, too, by having a cheerful person to care for him, one whose own needs are being met.

5. *The relative may need help from outsiders in caring for the patient.* Although the patient may object, the relative has the right to assess his own limitations of strength and endurance and to obtain assistance when required.

6. *The relative has a right to expect mutual consideration.* The world goes on, in spite of terminal illness and death. Therefore, mutual consideration between the patient and his relative must be worked for. When the relative knows that he is already doing all that can reasonably be expected of him in caring for the patient, he can have a clear conscience in maintaining contacts with the rest of the world. If the patient attempts to use illness as a weapon, the relative has the right to reject it.

7. *The relative has the right to feel himself free from responsibility for the patient's actions.* Since the patient has the right to make his own decisions regarding the course of illness (such as whether to take a nap, whether to take a pill, whether or not to seek unorthodox treatment), the relative must accept this independence of the patient. The patient's right to privacy and freedom of action can liberate the relative from burdensome con-

cerns. Though the relative may feel hurt at times because his earnest offer of help is rejected, he should realize that the patient still needs normal feelings of independence.

If someone thinks he or his relatives are being denied any of their rights, he should speak up—communicate with the doctor, nurses, and administrators.

BILL OF RIGHTS FOR NURSING HOMES AND CONVALESCENT CENTERS

Another area of concern in the health-care industry is that of nursing homes and convalescent centers. These facilities care for the elderly and ill who do not need hospitalization but who perhaps are not able to live alone. For such people, nursing homes and convalescent centers have come into prominence. The residents of these centers have certain rights also. The Department of Health and Human Resources has drafted a Bill of Rights[3] that requires these facilities to promote and protect each resident's rights as a citizen to dignified existence, self-determination, communication, and access to persons and services inside and outside the facility. The document provides the patient:

1. *Exercise of rights.* [The patient] may expect his/her rights, pursue interests, recommend changes in policy or service and voice grievances without restraint, interference, coercion, discrimination, or reprisal.

[The patient] may expect that all rights and responsibilities will devolve to the legal guardian, next of kin, or sponsoring agency, or the representative payee, when a resident is adjudicated incompetent and the attending physician finds the resident medically incapable of understanding these rights or has a communication barrier.

[The patient] may expect that an elderly person (fifty-five years of age or older) may not be denied appropriate care on the basis of race, religion, color, national origin, sex, age, handicap, marital status, or source of payment.

[The patient] may expect not to be prohibited from communicating in a national language with others for the purpose of acquiring or providing any type of treatment, care, or service.

2. *Freedom of Association.* [The resident] may expect to receive visitors and to associate freely inside or outside the facility with persons of his/her choice unless to do so would infringe upon the rights of others, and unless medically contraindicated (as documented by his/her physician). If married, [the resident] may expect to be assured privacy for visits by his/her spouse. If both are residents of the facility, they are permitted to share a room unless medically contraindicated as documented by his/her physician in the medical record.

3. *Access to Facility.* [The resident] may expect that the resident's representative and representatives of any federally mandated ombudsman will be allowed to the resident during normal visiting hours or as required by the resident.

4. *Resident Council.* [The resident] may expect the facility to allow the formation of a Resident Council by interested residents. And [they may expect] that residents will be assisted to meetings as required.

5. *Privacy.* [The resident] may expect the facility to ensure the resident's right to privacy in the following areas:

   a. *Accommodations.* Living quarters will provide privacy when caring for personal needs.

   b. *Medical treatment.* The facility will provide privacy to residents during examinations, treatment, case discussions, and consultations.

   c. *Telephone.* The facility will provide at least one telephone for resident use. The telephone will be in an accessible location and be available to residents at all times. Residents will be allowed to contract for private telephones to be connected to a central switchboard.

   d. *Mail.* The facility will not open or read residents' incoming or outgoing mail without their written permission. An individual's mail may not be opened unless authorized in writing by a physician. If requested by a resident, the facility will help open and read incoming mail and help address and post outgoing mail.

   6. *Confidentiality of Records.* [The resident] may expect the facility to maintain the confidentiality of a resident's personal and medical records and refuse their release to any individual outside the facility without the resident's written consent, except in the case of transfer to another facility, during Medicare or Medicaid surveys, or as otherwise required by law or third-party payment contracts. The facility will hold in confidence all matters related to the treatment, examination, case discussion, or consultation of the resident. An elderly individual may inspect his/her personal records (fifty-five years or older).

   7. *Property.* [The resident] may expect to retain his/her personal property and possessions as space permits. Limitations of possessions as due to health and safety reasons will be documented in the resident's medical record.

   8. *Right to Manage Personal Funds.* [The resident] may expect the facility to allow the resident to manage his/her own personal funds, to designate another person to manage them, or to authorize in writing the facility to hold, safeguard, and account for his/her personal funds.

   9. *Protection of Funds.* [The resident] may expect to be fully informed in writing of all services provided by the facility and of any related charges including all charges for services not covered under Title XVIII or XIX of the

Social Security Act, or not covered by the monthly vendor rate.

[The resident] understands that his/her right to nursing home services is not contingent upon contributions.

[The resident] may select how his personal funds will be handled and is under no obligation to deposit funds with the facility. [He/She] may expect to be given reasonable access to his/her financial records.

[The resident] may expect the facility to provide a written statement at least quarterly to each resident, representative payee or responsible party.

10. *Transfers.* [The resident] may expect that if changes should occur in his/her physical or mental condition necessitating services or care which cannot be adequately provided by the facility, he/she will be transferred to an appropriate facility.

[The resident] may expect to be transferred only for medical reasons, or for his/her welfare or that of other residents, or for nonpayment for his/her stay (except where prohibited by Title XVIII or XIX of the Social Security Act).

[The resident] may expect, except for emergencies, the facility to notify in writing the resident, responsible party, and attending physician at least five (5) days before a transfer or discharge.

[The resident] may expect that if one's spouse wishes to transfer, the facility will give both married persons a notice of their rights to transfer to the same facility.

11. *Care Involvement.* [The resident] may expect the facility to accept or retain only persons whose needs can be met by the facility directly, or in cooperation with community resources, or other health care providers with which it is affiliated or has contracts.

[The resident] may expect to be treated with consideration, respect, and full recognition of his/her dignity.

[The resident] may expect to choose his/her own physician.

[The resident] may expect to be fully informed by a physician of his/her medical condition and have questions answered concerning his/her health treatment and condition, unless medically contraindicated (as documented in the medical record).

[The resident] is afforded the opportunity to participate in the planning of his/her medical treatment.

[The resident] is afforded the opportunity to refuse treatment and medications for other than religious reasons, and to be informed by his physician of the consequences of the decision to refuse treatment and medications.

[The resident] may expect the facility to respect the religious beliefs of the residents.

[The resident] has the right to refuse participation in any experimental research.

12. *Restraints.* [The resident] may expect to be free from mental and physical abuse and free from chemical and physical restraint except when authorized in writing by a physician for a specified and limited period of time, or when necessary in an emergency to protect the resident from injury to himself or to others.

[The resident] may expect that this facility will not physically or mentally abuse or exploit recipient-patients and elderly individuals or subject them to corporal punishment.

[The resident] may expect that the facility will not restrain or reimpose a restraint except upon the written order of a physician.

[The resident] may expect that residents who are physically or chemically restrained will be observed for complications and/or side effects.

[The resident] may expect a mentally retarded elderly individual to participate in a behavior modification program involving use of restraints or adverse stimuli only with the informed consent of a guardian.

13. *Statement of Services and Bills.* [The resident] may

expect to be fully informed in writing of all facility services and related charges, including any extra charges
for services not covered under Medicare and Medicaid
or daily rate.

[The resident] may expect that the facility will notify
him/her or a responsible party in advance of any
changes in rates or services not covered by Medicaid.

[The resident] may expect that he/she will be allowed freedom of choice in obtaining any Medicaid services from qualified providers except when the provider
causes the facility to be out of compliance with the
Department of Human Resources Standards of Participation.

14. *Religious Activities.* [The resident] may expect to
participate in activities of social, religious, and community groups at their discretion unless medically contraindicated for reasons documented in the medical
record by a physician.

[The resident] may expect requests by residents to see
specific members of the clergy to be honored and that
privacy will be provided.

15. *Acknowledgment of Rights.* [The resident] may
expect to be fully informed prior to or at time of admis-
sion to this facility of his/her rights and responsibilities
as a resident, and of all rules and regulations governing
resident conduct and responsibilities. A receipt from the
resident, guardian, or receipt with third-person witness
in the case of the mentally retarded individual, ac-
knowledging awareness of rights, responsibilities, conduct, rules, and regulations will be complete.

TWO
THE LIVING WILL
AND THE DYING
PATIENT'S RIGHTS

The so-called Living Will is a document representing the patient's intentions to be respected as one factor in considering his total health care. Some states have now passed specific legislative acts that have a bearing upon the rights of the terminally ill patient.

The main point of the Living Will is to express the personal desires of the patient to the family and health-care professionals. The following is an example of the form a Living Will might take:

A Living Will to my family, my physician, my lawyer,.
and all others whom it may concern:
Death is as much a reality as birth, growth, and maturity, and old age—it is the one certainty of life. If the time comes when I can no longer take part in decisions for my own future, let this statement, made while I am still of sound mind, stand as an expression of my wishes and directions:

If at such a time the situation should arise in which there is no reasonable expectation of my recovery from extreme physical or mental disability, I direct that I be allowed to die and not to be kept alive by medications, artificial means, or "heroic measures." I do, however, ask that medication be mercifully administered to me to alleviate suffering even though such medication may shorten my remaining life.

This statement is made after careful consideration and is in accordance with my strong conviction and beliefs. I want the wishes and directions here expressed carried out to the extent permitted by law. Insofar as they are not legally enforceable, I hope that those to whom this Will is addressed will regard themselves as morally bound by these provisions.

To make best use of the Living Will, the writer should:

1. Sign and date it before two witnesses. (This is to assure that it is signed of the writer's own free will and that he is not under any pressure.)

2. If a doctor is already engaged, he should have a copy of the medical file, and the Living Will agreement should be discussed with him.

Copies of the Living Will should be given to all of those people who are most likely to be concerned with the phrase "if the time comes when I can no longer take part in decisions for my own future." Their names should be entered on the bottom line of the Living Will. The original of it should be kept nearby, easily and readily available.

3. Above all, the one who makes a Living Will should discuss all his intentions with those who are closest to him, NOW.

4. It is a good idea to look over the Living Will once a year, redate it, and initial the new date to make it clear that the intentions of the one who made it are unchanged.

Declarants may see the importance of adding specific statements to the Living Will to be inserted in the space provided for that purpose above the signature. Possible additional provisions might be any or all of the below:

1. a. I appoint _____
      to make binding decisions concerning my medi-
      cal treatment, OR
   b. I have discussed my views as to life-sustaining
      measures with the following who understand
      my wishes:

   _____

   _____

   _____

2. Measures of artificial life support in the face of impending death that are especially abhorrent to me are:
   a. Electrical or mechanical resuscitation of my
      heart when it has stopped beating.
   b. Nasogastric tube feedings when I am paralyzed
      and no longer able to swallow.
   c. Mechanical respiration by machine when my
      brain can no longer sustain my own breathing.
   d. _____ .

3. If it does not jeopardize the chance of my recovery
to a meaningful and sentient life or impose an undue
burden on my family, I would like to live out my last
days at home rather than in a hospital.

4. If any of my tissues are sound and would be of
value as transplants to help other people, I freely give
my permission for such donation.

Signed _____

Date _____

Witness _____

_____

35

Copies of this request have been given to ⎯⎯⎯⎯⎯⎯

⎯⎯⎯⎯⎯⎯⎯⎯⎯⎯⎯⎯⎯⎯⎯⎯⎯⎯⎯⎯⎯⎯⎯⎯⎯⎯⎯⎯⎯⎯⎯⎯⎯

⎯⎯⎯⎯⎯⎯⎯⎯⎯⎯⎯⎯⎯⎯⎯⎯⎯⎯⎯⎯⎯⎯⎯⎯⎯⎯⎯⎯⎯⎯⎯⎯⎯

There are some questions about the Living Will, most entailing the greater question "Is the document legally binding and enforceable?"

The Living Will is an advisory document that is legally binding and enforceable to the extent that the patient's wishes are formally stated in writing. Therefore, if any legal, medical, or ethical questions arise concerning care and treatment, there is no doubt as to the desires of the person. Since the courts are ultimately concerned with the patient's own wishes, the properly drafted and executed declaration of the Living Will, stating desires prior to any incompetence or coma, should permit the health-care professionals to follow the patient's wishes without going to court for personal immunity. Ultimately this is usually a very private matter, dealt with by the physician and family member responsible for the patient. Upon making a Living Will, one should promptly discuss it with family, physician, and attorney. Copies of the Living Will should be filed along with other important papers, but copies should be easily accessible to all people concerned, such as next of kin, physicians, attorneys, and ministers. Since there may arise at any time an immediate need for it, it should not be filed away in a place where it will not be located until it is too late.

THE DYING PERSON'S BILL OF RIGHTS

Someone who realizes he is dying has certain human rights as a dying person. In our society, the dying person, whether he looks ill or not, is often avoided or in other ways stigmatized. The general public has a tendency to relate to the dying in a superficial manner because they do not know what to say or not to say. As a result, impolite or rude behavior is too often tolerated. Dying people then feel even more isolated and lonely. They become unable to relate their fears and feelings with their relatives and friends as to how to make realistic plans for the future.

The following self-explanatory list describes the dying person's rights.[1]

1. I have the right to be treated as a living human being until I die.

2. I have the right to maintain a sense of hopefulness, however changing its focus may be.

3. I have the right to be cared for by those who can maintain a sense of hopefulness, however changing this might be.

4. I have the right to express in my own way my feelings and emotions about my approaching death.

5. I have the right to participate in decisions concerning my care.

6. I have the right to expect continuing medical and nursing attention, even though "cure" goals must be changed to "comfort" goals.

7. I have the right not to die alone.

8. I have the right to be free from pain.

9. I have the right to have my questions answered honestly.

10. I have the right not to be deceived.

11. I have the right to have help from and for my family in accepting my death.

12. I have the right to die in peace and dignity.

13. I have the right to retain my individuality and not to be judged for my decisions, which may be contrary to beliefs of others.

14. I have the right to discuss and enlarge my religious and spiritual experiences.

15. I have the right to expect that the sanctity of the human body will be respected after death.

16. I have the right to be cared for by caring, sensitive, knowledgeable people who will attempt to understand my needs and will be able to gain some satisfaction in helping me face my death.

As the dying person realizes certain "rights," then he needs some insights into living with a terminal illness, which will be discussed in the following chapter.

THREE
LIVING WITH
TERMINAL ILLNESS

Although there have been great advancements in the medical world, people are still being diagnosed as terminally ill. The question arises, "What happens between the time a person finds out he is terminally ill and the time he actually dies?"

The greatest difference between the terms *acutely dying* and *chronically dying* is the estimated time spent in the span of dying. The chronically dying person may take several months or years before dying. He may even reach plateaus of various degrees of wellness, but he knows from the diagnosis that he is terminally ill. The acutely ill person may have only a few hours, days, or weeks to live. He may not have the opportunity to work through all the issues that the chronically ill person may have.

Yet, time for the chronically dying person is a two-edged sword. The positive side gives him the luxury of being with family and time to fulfill some of his goals as he experiences the last days on earth. The negative side represents his diminished abilities, pain, loneliness, and the grief of leaving his loved ones.

Some terminally ill people feel that they have too much time. Once they know they are going to die in the near future, they would just as soon get it over with. During their prolonged wait, they experience boredom, decreased communication and social skills, strained family relationships, negative self-image, and even physical deterioration. Most of these people just exist in gloomy sadness that life is coming to a close. It does not have to be that way! Orville Kelly, the founder of Make Today Count,[1] has developed ten self-explanatory suggestions to help people to live with a terminal illness. These suggestions should be read slowly and then discussed with family and friends.

SUGGESTIONS FOR THE TERMINALLY ILL

1. Talk about the illness. Call the illness by its name. If it is cancer, call it cancer. You cannot make life normal again by trying to hide what is wrong.

2. Accept death as a part of life. It is!

3. Consider each day as another day of life, a gift from God to be enjoyed as fully as possible.

4. Realize that life is never going to be perfect. It was not before, and it will not be now.

5. Pray. It is not a sign of weakness. It is your strength.

6. Learn to live with your illness instead of considering yourself as dying from it. We are all dying in some manner.

7. Put your friends and relatives at ease yourself. If you do not want pity, do not ask for it.

8. Make all practical arrangements for memorial services, funerals, wills, etc., and make certain your family understands them.

9. Set new goals; realize your limitations. Sometimes the simple things of life become the most enjoyable.

10. Discuss your problems with your family as they occur. Include the children if possible. After all, your problem is not an individual one.

THE CHRISTIAN AFFIRMATION OF LIFE

The Christian Affirmation of Life[2] is a statement developed to assist people who are living with terminal illness. It expresses a faith in God by the patient to all who are caring for him.

To my family, friends, physician, lawyer, and clergyman: I believe that each individual person is created by God our Father in love and that God retains a loving relationship to each person throughout human life and eternity.

I believe that Jesus Christ lived, suffered, and died for me and that his suffering, death, and resurrection prefigure and make possible the death-resurrection process which I now anticipate.

I believe that each person's worth and dignity derive from the relationship of love in Christ that God has for each individual person and not from one's usefulness or effectiveness in society.

I believe that God our Father has entrusted to me a shared dominion with him over my earthly existence so that I am bound to use ordinary means to preserve my life but I am free to refuse extraordinary means to prolong my life.

I believe that through death life is not taken away but merely changed, and though I may experience fear, suffering, and sorrow, by the grace of the Holy Spirit I hope to accept death as a free human act that enables me to surrender this life and to be united with God for eternity.

Because of my belief:

I, _____, request that I be informed as death approaches so that I may continue to prepare for the full encounter with Christ through the

41

help of the sacraments and the consolation and prayers of my family and friends.

I request that, if possible, I be consulted concerning the medical procedures which might be used to prolong my life as death approaches. If I can no longer take part in decisions concerning my own future and there is no reasonable expectation of my recovery from physical and mental disability, I request that no extraordinary means be used to prolong my life.

I request, though I wish to join my suffering to the suffering of Jesus so I may be united fully with him in the act of death-resurrection, that my pain, if unbearable, be alleviated. However, no means should be used with the intention of shortening my life.

I request, because I am a sinner and in need of reconciliation and because my faith, hope, and love may not overcome all fear and doubt, that my family, friends, and the whole Christian community join me in prayer and mortification as I prepare for the great personal act of dying.

Finally, I request that after my death, my family, my friends and the whole Christian community rejoice with me because of the mercy and love of the Trinity, with whom I hope to be united for eternity.

Signed _____

REFUSAL OF CONSENT

Many terminally ill people are living more psychologically comfortable lives since signing a refusal to consent for life-prolonging procedures. The following is an example of such a document.

Refusal of Consent for Life-prolonging Procedures

To any and all doctors, hospitals, health personnel, and others treating me during my final illness:

I, _____, hereby make this statement in the presence of witnesses, to declare and record my express wish and desire that: In the event, due to illness or accident, that my condition becomes terminal and without reasonable hope of recovery, then I do not wish to be kept alive by the use of drugs, treatments, or machine. I wish to receive adequate medications for proper control of my symptoms, but nothing beyond what is necessary for that purpose. I hereby specifically withdraw my consent for any such primarily life-sustaining treatment, and this withdrawal of my consent shall continue unless and until I revoke it in writing. Should I, in the course of my illness, subsequently become legally incompetent or unable to communicate my wishes to those treating me, then this document should be considered as continuing to withdraw my consent to any further treatment not directed primarily at symptom relief. Any and all doctors, nurses, hospitals, and institutions that honor my wishes and intentions as expressed in this document are hereby formally held free from any and all liability on behalf of myself, my heirs, successors, and assigns.

Signed _____

Date _____

Witnesses _____

_____

THE TEN COMMANDMENTS ABOUT DEATH

Impending death is not only a difficult time for the person dying but also for the family and friends. In that period of time, while a person is dying, the people around can be of significant help. There are ten commandments for dealing with death.[3]

1. *Tell the patient that he is dying.* Regardless of the age of the dying person, he should have complete knowledge about his condition. This is important, since

sooner or later he will discover the truth anyway.

2. *Be aware of the emotional stages the dying person normally experiences.* Dr. Elizabeth Kubler-Ross pioneered the description of the stages of grief (as discussed in chapter 8), which she outlined as denial, anger, bargaining, depression, and acceptance.

3. *Do not isolate the dying person.* Most dying people relate that their greatest fear is not of dying itself, but of dying alone. In American and Canadian societies, death has been such a forbidden topic of discussion that even the medical personnel have had some unhealthy attitudes about it. It seems that we want to get the dying person far away from the living so the living will not have to face realities.

4. *Talk about dying with the terminally ill patient.* It is extremely rare that a dying person does not desire to discuss his illness and dying. People need to understand what is happening to their physically debilitated body. Perhaps it will seem awkward at first, but soon communication can move toward being something that is gratifying for all people involved.

5. *Encourage the dying person to talk about his fears.* A dying person develops anxieties and fears that may become distorted completely out of proportion. Open communication is often the key to alleviating many problems that the dying encounter.

6. *Treat the dying person as a person.* A dying person has self-value, dignity, worth—just as a physically healthy person. The dying person should not be *treated* like an invalid or a child. The dying need to be included in decisions that affect the family and friends.

7. *Do not be afraid to make plans.* Whatever the dying person desires to talk about, be open and permit complete communication. The dying should be permitted to talk about wills, funerals, and plans for family. The dying person should know that he may reopen the discussions at any time he desires.

8. *Do things now—tomorrow may be too late.* For a dying person, each day counts. He feels a great sense of urgency. Sometimes it is not necessarily the "big things" that count so much as the "little things." The dying are more comfortable trying to do everything right now. Spending this kind of time with the dying may produce some very pleasant memories for everyone involved.

9. *Encourage the dying person to maintain a feeling of hope.* A good attitude and positive mental perspective may do more to prolong life than can any particular medicine. In other words, patient and family should stop counting time and make time count!

10. *Look to the dying person's faith in God for some ultimate sense of order.* The dying person and his family and friends can draw great strength from the Scriptures. The friends and family should give affirmation to faith in God. We can draw deep meaning from the truth that we do not know how to live until we know how to die. There is a practical realistic way in which one can decide to keep on living with terminal illness. The following is a contract someone can make with himself to organize and make his time more meaningful.

Contract with Myself
I contract with myself to choose to keep on living until I die. I will daily work on the following.
I. Personal Goals
  A. Immediate (1 to 6 weeks) I will _____

_____

_____

  B. Long range (6 weeks to 6 months) I will _____

_____

_____

II. Personal planning
I will take the following action steps to reach my goals:

A. _____

B. _____

C. _____

D. _____

E. _____

III. Personal Thoughts and Feelings
   Thoughts

Positive (helpful)	Negative (nonhelpful)
A. _____	A. _____
B. _____	B. _____
C. _____	C. _____
D. _____	D. _____
E. _____	E. _____

   Feelings

Positive (helpful)	Negative (nonhelpful)
A. _____	A. _____
B. _____	B. _____
C: _____	C. _____
D. _____	D. _____
E. _____	E. _____

IV. Personal Rewards
If I complete my goals I will reward myself in the following ways:

A. _____

B. _____

C. _____

D. _____

E. _____

V. Personal Cost
If I do not complete my goals I will ask myself to do the following:

A. _____

B. _____

C. _____

D. _____

E. _____

VI. Reevaluation
As I reevaluate the short- and long-range goals, I find the following:

A. _____

B. _____

C. _____

D. _____

E. _____

VII. Support System
   A. I agree to be a support person:

   _____

   (signature of a support person)
   B. I agree to strive toward this contract with myself:

   _____

   (your signature)

As the dying person is learning to live with a terminal illness, he may need to deal with pain control, which will be discussed in the next chapter.

FOUR
PAIN CONTROL

For a person enduring severe pain, release is the only thing that really matters. Pain, whether physical, emotional, or a combination, depletes the energies of the body and mind. The pleasant things of life lose their meaning when pain is more distracting than anything else. A constant raging war going on within a person's nervous system affects the reasoning center, energy level, and one's spiritual status. Pain often seems to permeate a person's total being.

Pain is a response to a specific stimulus. It usually causes us to desire to communicate with other people. One of my friends says, "Anyone who says, 'I am in pain' wants a response from another person." This person's conscious motive may be inconsistent with his unconscious desire. Some people may be wanting attention by indirectly communicating, "Poor me, I am suffering so much," or perhaps, "See how wonderful I am as I endure the pain?" Both are attempts to use their pain to manipulate other people.

Everyone has experienced some pain—from a cut finger, a stubbed toe, or a headache. Such pain is predictable and tolerated well by most people. Pain from a terminal illness or a serious injury, for which the duration is unpredictable, is less well tolerated.

Since no two people experience pain in the same way, it is unlikely that any two injuries or illnesses would create identical responses. For some people in pain, total relief never comes and interventions are required to minimize the pain. The interpretation and meaning of pain involves several cultural, psychological, as well as physiological factors, since pain, being highly subjective, cannot be objectively determined and measured.

Some types of pain do create predictable signs and symptoms. For a long time, researchers thought that everyone perceived pain the same way. Pain threshold is usually defined as the point at which a person first perceives a stimulus as painful. An individual's pain threshold is mainly related to his physiology, yet psychological, emotional, and spiritual influences can affect the way someone labels something as being painful.

Medical researchers have revealed that the higher centers of the central nervous system work together to perceive the onset of pain and its nature and significance. Perception of the pain is influenced by the cerebral cortex. Thus, the pain we feel is affected by past experiences, values, emotions, and physical characteristics.

Since pain perception includes values and manner in which pain should be expressed, a person's behavior is drastically affected. If someone thinks pain is a punishment or personal weakness, he will probably not express any discomfort. If a person thinks the pain is undeserved or unwarranted, then he is usually more open about expression.

In our culture we learn expectations about the significance and meaning of pain. Young children learn quickly that certain behavioral responses are rewarded with pleasure or punished with pain. Thus, emotions have an influential role in pain perception. If we feel happy and involved in activities, there is no time to dwell on moderate discomfort. But if we are depressed or lonely, we will concentrate on discomfort and our pain perceptions are greater.

Responses to pain are very different. Our tolerance to pain refers to the point at which we are unwilling to accept pain of any greater severity or duration. The patient who has a high pain tolerance can endure periods of severe pain without assistance. In order to keep a positive self-image the patient minimizes his responses to the pain. As time goes by, fatigue will lessen the time it takes for him to react to painful stimuli. Then his energy level falls and pain is less tolerable, but he can still get rest.

On the other hand, the patient who has a low pain tolerance will probably try to get relief before the pain heightens. This person may request medication in anticipation even before the pain gets intense. Pain, then, is a complex series of physical, psychological, emotional, and spiritual responses.

Pain, as we have said, is labeled either as acute or chronic. At what point acute pain becomes chronic pain is relative. Acute pain is brief in duration and an end is anticipated. Chronic pain lasts over a prolonged period of time and most patients never get complete relief. Chronic pain seems to be timeless, endless, and meaningless. Many people make pain even worse by anticipating it.

The medical professionals have studied pain control at great length. In the last few years, research has produced some significant information about the mechanisms by which the human body generates and suppresses pain. Both chemical and nonchemical methods of treatment of pain have been more fully developed. Understanding and coping with pain involves dealing with biological, psychological, procedural, spiritual, and moral questions. Some hard-to-answer questions are these:

1. When can pain be eliminated?
2. When can pain be controlled?
3. What are chemical and drug treatments?
4. What are nonchemical treatments?
5. When is treatment worse than the disease?
6. When is it appropriate to give addictive drugs?
7. How does the patient's negative or positive attitude affect his pain?
8. What about the debilitating effect pain has on the emotions and spirit?
9. How should one relate to a patient whose pain has exhausted his ability to reciprocate warmth or affection?
10. Where are the most recognized hospitals for controlling pain?

The answers to these questions are not easy. Managing chronic pain is one of the greatest problems posed to medical science. Pain that has persisted for long periods of time can erode the physical body, personality, family life, and social relationships. Since it is not possible for anyone to live completely free from pain, a person's attitude toward pain is directly linked to one's attitude toward reality.

Physicians usually agree that acute pain becomes chronic pain when it lasts more than six months. There are four major methods to treat pain:

1. *Chemical or drug therapy,* the use of mild to heavy drugs, usually analgesic agents for treatment of specific symptoms.

2. *Physical methods,* such as nerve blocks and sometimes the use of transcutaneous electrical nerve stimulation, sometimes called TENS (a controlled flow of low voltage through the skin and outer tissues to stimulate nerve endings).

3. *Psychiatric therapy or psychotherapy* to help the

patient adjust and deal with his pain. Biofeedback, a technique of retraining the mind to react to pain stimulus, has become an effective pain control measure.

4. *Psychosomatic treatment* to deal with specific psychological abnormalities.

PAIN CONTROL

The consensus of medical opinion seems to be that pain control should take the following course:

1. Begin with non-narcotic analgesics.
2. Respect individual differences among people.
3. Administer the mild analgesics on a regular basis.
4. If necessary, use a combination of effective drugs.
5. Anticipate some side effects.
6. Observe the patient for the tolerance level.
7. Withdraw the medication slowly.
8. Continue heavier drugs only when there is no other alternative.

Trying to describe pain is as impossible as trying to describe a beautiful western sunset to a blind person. There are no words or concepts that are appropriate because pain is so personal and variable.

Pain should sometimes be considered as something positive. It can serve as a warning signal that something is wrong with the physical body. Yet, there is the devastating and negative side to pain. Many diseases attack without pain warning. Then, when the patient feels the pain, perhaps it is already too late for medical science to heal him. Pain is also a protective mechanism. It can be a warning that damage is occurring. Therefore, anyone in pain should seek medical attention.

Although there have been many advances in the medical field concerning pain control, experts admit that whereas they were in the basement of dealing with chronic pain, they are now perhaps on the ground-floor level.

PAIN CLINICS

It may be desirable to seek professional help in the control of pain. Some pain clinics have gained widespread acceptance. A patient usually has to be referred to the pain clinic by a physician. The following is a comprehensive list of pain clinics in the United States:

Alabama
Pain Clinic
1029 Christine
Anniston, AL 36201

University of Alabama in Birmingham
19th Street, 6th Avenue, South
Birmingham, AL 36201

Arizona
Surgicenter Pain Control Unit
1040 East McDowell
Phoenix, AZ 85010

Tucson Medical Center
Tanque Verde Anesthesia, Ltd.
Ambulatory Surgical Center
Tuscon, AZ 85702

University of Arizona Pain Clinic
1501 North Campbell Avenue
Tucson, AZ 85717

Veterans Hospital
Tucson, AZ 85717

California
Biofeedback Medical Clinic
9735 Wilshire Boulevard
Beverly Hills, CA 90213

The Chinese Acupuncture Therapy for Pain
Carson Medical Center
Carson, CA 90744

Rancho Los Amigos Hospital
Spine Center
7601 East Imperial Highway
Downey, CA 90241

Pain Center
City of Hope National Medical Center
1500 East Duarte Road
Duarte, CA 91010

Pain Treatment Center
Scripps Clinic Medical Institutions
10666 North Torrey Pines Road
La Jolla, CA 92037

Pain Control Center
Loma Linda University Medical Center
Loma Linda, CA 92354

Naval Regional Medical Center
7500 East Caron Street
Long Beach, CA 90801

Anesthesiology and Pain Management
1300 North Vermont Avenue
Los Angeles, CA 90052

Pain Center
UCLA School of Medicine
Los Angeles, CA 90007

University of Southern California
School of Dentistry
TMJ and Peri-Oral Pain Clinic
925 West 34th Street
Los Angeles, CA 90052

Veterans Administration Wadsworth Hospital
Santelle and Wilshire Boulevard
Los Angeles, CA 90025

El Camino Hospital
Mountain View, CA 94040

Pain Control Medical Group
7535 Laurel Canyon Boulevard
North Hollywood, CA 90028

Huntington Memorial Hospital
Pain Clinic
100 Congress Street
Pasadena, CA 91109

Casa Colina Hospital
for Rehabilitation Medicine
255 East Bonita Avenue
Pomona, CA 91766

University of California
Davis-Sacramento Medical Center
4301 "X" Street
Sacramento, CA 95813

Mercy Hospital and Medical Center
4077 5th Avenue
San Diego, CA 92101

Naval Regional Medical Center
San Diego, CA 92134

Veterans Administration Hospital
3350 La Jolla Village Drive
San Diego, CA 92101

Department of Anesthesia
University of California
San Francisco, CA 94101

Letterman Army Medical Center
San Francisco, CA 94101

Medical Center
University of California
San Francisco, CA 94101

Veterans Administration Hospital
4150 Clement Street
San Francisco, CA 94101

Cox Pain Center
2066-B Chorro Street
San Luis Obispo, CA 93401

James Y. P. Chen, M.D.
1304 15th Street
Santa Monica, CA 90406

St. John's Hospital
1238 22nd Street
Santa Monica, CA 90406

Stanford University Medical Center
Anesthesia Department
Nerve Block Clinic
Stanford, CA 94305

Harbor General Hospital Pain Clinic
Harbor General Hospital
1000 West Carson Street
Torrance, CA 90510

Southwest Surgical Clinic
4201 Torrance Boulevard,
Suite 240
Torrance, CA 90503

Colorado
Pain Clinic
University of Colorado Medical Center
Denver, CO 80202

St. Joseph's Hospital
Denver, CO 80202

Veterans Administration Hospital
Denver, CO 80202

U. S. Army Hospital
Fort Carson, CO 80913

Connecticut
Pain Clinic
Greenwich Hospital
Perryridge Road
Greenwich, CT 06830

Research Institute of Acupuncture
and Chinese Medicine
North Benson Road
Middlebury, CT 06762

Veterans Administration Hospital
West Haven, CT 06516

District of Columbia
Georgetown Hospital
Washington, DC 20007

Greater Southeast Community Hospital
1310 Southern Avenue, S.E.
Washington, DC 20013

Providence Hospital
Washington, DC 20013

Florida
Mt. Sinai Pain Center
Mt. Sinai Medical Center of Greater Miami
Gainesville, FL 32601

Pain Control
Department of Anesthesiology
Shands Teaching Hospital
University of Florida
Gainesville, FL 32601

University of Florida
College of Dentistry
Gainesville, FL 32601

University of Miami School of Medicine
Department of Neurosurgery
Gainesville, FL 32601

Veterans Administration Hospital
Gainesville, FL 32601

Fish Memorial Hospital
401 Palmetto Street
New Smyrna Beach, FL 32069

Naval Aerospace Regional
Medical Center
Pensacola, FL 32508

W. C. Payne Medical Arts Building
5149 North 9th Avenue
Suite 307
Pensacola, FL 32502

Hubert Rutland Hospital
5115 58th Avenue, North
St. Petersburg, FL 33730

Georgia
Emory Pain Control Center
Emory University Center of Rehabilitation Medicine
Atlanta, GA 30333

Georgia Baptist Medical Center
300 Boulevard
Atlanta, GA 30304

Atlanta Pain Clinic
2550 Windy Hill Road
Suite 104
Marietta, GA 30060

Idaho
St. Joseph's Hospital
Pain Clinic
Lewistown, ID 83501

Illinois
Central Community Hospital
5701 South Wood Street
Chicago, IL 60607

Cook County Hospital
1825 West Harrison Street
Chicago, IL 60607

Diamond Headache Clinic, Ltd.
5252 North Western Avenue
Chicago, IL 60607

Illinois Masonic Medical Center
836 Wellington
Chicago, IL 60607

Low Back and Pain Clinic
Northwestern University Medical Center
Chicago, IL 60607

Michael Reese Medical Center
29th at Ellis Avenue
Chicago, IL 60607

Rush Pain Center
1725 West Harrison Street
Suite 262
Chicago, IL 60607

Schwab Rehabilitation Hospital
1401 South California Boulevard
Chicago, IL 60607

Thorek Medical Center and Hospital
850 West Irving Park Road
Chicago, IL 60607

Temporomandibular Joint and Facial Pain
Research Center
University of Illinois
College of Dentistry
Chicago, IL 60607

University of Illinois Pain Clinic
840 South Wood Street
Chicago, IL 60607

North Chicago Veterans Administration Hospital
Downey, IL 60064

U. S. Naval Regional Medical Center
Great Lakes, IL 60088

Loyola University Hospital
2160 South First Avenue
Maywood, IL 60153

Delnor Hospital
St. Charles, IL 60174

R. C. Balagot, M.D., and Associates, Ltd.
4332 Oakton Street
Skokie, IL 60076

Marianjoy Rehabilitation Hospital
Wheaton, IL 60187

Indiana
Elkhart General Hospital
Elkhart, IN 46514

St. Mary Medical Center
540 Tyler Street
Gary, IN 46401

Community Hospital
Rehabilitation Center for Pain
Indianapolis, IN 46206

St. Joseph's Hospital
South Bend, IN 46624

Iowa
St. Joseph Mercy Hospital
Mason City, IA 50401

Neurological Institute and Pain Center
809 Badgerow Building
Sioux City, IA 51101

Kentucky
Pain Rehabilitation Clinic
University of Kentucky Medical Center
Lexington, KY 40201

University of Louisville Pain Clinic
316 MDR Building
Health Science Center
Louisville, KY 40201

Veterans Hospital Pain Clinic
Louisville, KY 40201

Louisiana
Pain Clinic—New Orleans
3225 North Labarre Road
Metairie, LA 70004

Doctor's Hospital Pain Unit
Doctor's Hospital
Shreveport, LA 71102

Maine
Maine Medical Center
22 Bramhall Street
Portland, ME 04101

Maryland
Baltimore City Hospital
4940 Eastern Avenue
Baltimore, MD 21233

Pain Treatment Center
Johns Hopkins Hospital
601 North Broadway
Baltimore, MD 21233

Myo-Oral Facial Pain Clinic
University of Maryland School of Dentistry
Baltimore, MD 21233

University of Maryland Hospital
Baltimore, MD 21233

Associated Pain Consultants
8808 Cameron Street
Silver Spring, MD 20907

Fairland Pain Clinic
13616 Colefair Drive
Silver Spring, MD 20907

Mensana Clinic
Greenspring Valley Road
Stevenson, MD 21153

Massachusetts
Beth Israel Hospital
Harvard Medical School
Boston, MA 02109

Carney Hospital
2100 Dorchester Avenue
Boston, MA 02109

Pain Service
Massachusetts General Hospital
Fruit Street
Boston, MA 02109

Peter B. Brigham Hospital
125 Parker Hill Avenue
Boston, MA 02109

Kennedy Memorial Pediatric Hospital
30 Warren Street
Brighton, MA 02135

Baystate Medical Center
Chestnut Street
Springfield, MA 01101

New England Rehabilitation Hospital
Woburn, MA 01801

Pain Clinic
University of Massachusetts Medical Center
Worcester, MA 01601

Michigan
University of Michigan Medical Center
Ann Arbor, MI 48106

Sinai Hospital of Detroit
6767 West Outer Drive
Detroit, MI 48233

Ingham Medical Center Pain Clinic
401 West Greenlawn
Lansing, MI 48924

Detroit Pain Clinic
16800 West 12 Mile Road
Suite 203
Southfield, MI 48075

Rehabilitation Center
22401 Foster Winter Drive
Southfield, MI 48075

Minnesota
St. Joseph's Hospital
Mankato, MN 56001

Metropolitan Medical Center
and Waconia Ridgeview Hospital
Minneapolis, MN 55401

Minneapolis Pain Clinic
4225 Golden Valley Road
Minneapolis, MN 55401

Mount Sinai Hospital
2215 Park Avenue
Minneapolis, MN 55401

Pain Management Center
St. Mary's Hospital—Mayo Clinic
Minneapolis, MN 55401

Pain Clinic
Mayo Clinic
Rochester, MN 55901

St. Louis Park Treatment Center
3705 Park Center Boulevard
St. Louis Park, MN 55426

St. Paul Ramsey Hospital
and Medical Center
640 Jackson Street
St. Paul, MN 55101

Mississippi
Curtis W. Caine, M.D.
Jackson, MS 39205

Mississippi University Medical Center
2500 North State Street
Jackson, MS 39205

Jeff Anderson Hospital
Meridian, MS 39301

Missouri
Howard County General Chronic Pain Clinic
Cedar Lane and Little Patuxent Parkway
Columbia, MO 65201

Harry S. Truman Memorial Veterans
Administration Hospital
800 Stadium Boulevard
Columbia, MO 65201

University of Missouri Medical Center
Rusk Rehabilitation Center
Columbia, MO 65201

Victor M. Parisien, MOPA
416 Sabbatus Street
Lewiston, MO 63452

Montana
Missoula Pain Clinic
Missoula Community Hospital
Missoula, MT 59801

Nebraska
Nebraska Pain Rehabilitation Unit
University of Nebraska Medical Center
Omaha, NE 68108

The Pain Clinic
7701 Pacific Street
Suite 123
Omaha, NB 86108

New Hampshire
Dartmouth-Hitchcock Medical Center
Hanover, NH 03755

Cheshire Hospital
580 Court Street
Keene, NH 03431

New Jersey
Pain Clinic New Jersey Medical School
and Affiliated Hospitals
Newark, NJ 07102

St. Joseph's Hospital and Medical Center
703 Main Street
Paterson, NJ 07510

North Jersey Anesthesia Associates
220 Hamburg Turnpike
Wayne, NJ 07470

Kessler Institute of Rehabilitation
1199 Pleasant Valley Way
West Orange, NJ 07052

New Mexico
Lovelace Bataan Medical Center
5200 Gibson Boulevard
Albuquerque, NM 87101

New York
Our Lady of Lourdes Hospital
Pain Unit
169 Riverside Drive
Binghamton, NY 13904

Acupuncture Clinic
Revson Diagnostic Center
Hospital of the Albert Einstein College of Medicine
Bronx, NY 10451

Montefiore Hospital and Medical Center
Headache Unit
111 East 210th Street
Bronx, NY 10451

Maimonides Medical Center
Department of Anesthesiology
Brooklyn, NY 11201

Sisters of Charity Hospital
2157 Main Street
Buffalo, NY 13240

Parsons Acupuncture Clinic
Parsons Hospital
34-14 Parsons Boulevard
Flushing, NY 11351

Boulevard Hospital
46-04 31st Avenue
Long Island City, NY 11101

Facial Pain—Temporomandibular Joint Clinic
Columbia University
School of Dental and Oral Surgery
New York, NY 10025

Hospital for Joint Diseases and Medical Center
Pain Program
1919 Madison Avenue
New York, NY 10010

Memorial Sloan-Kettering Cancer Center
1275 York Avenue
New York, NY 10001

Nerve Block Clinic and Neurology Clinic
Presbyterian Hospital
Vanderbilt Clinic
Columbia-Presbyterian Medical Center
Broadway and 168th Street
New York, NY 10025

New York Hospital
Cornell University Medical Center
525 East 68th Street
New York, NY 10023

Phelps Memorial Hospital
North Tarrytown, NY 10591

Strong Memorial Hospital
601 Elmwood Avenue
Rochester, NY 14603

S.U.N.Y. Upstate Medical Center
750 East Adams Street
Syracuse, NY 13210

Pain Clinic
Westchester County Medical Center
Valhalla, NY 10595

North Carolina
University of North Carolina Pain Clinic
North Carolina Memorial Hospital
and Dental Research Center
Chapel Hill, NC 27514

Pain Clinic
Duke University Medical Center
Durham, NC 27706

Ohio
Cincinnati General Hospital
Cincinnati, OH 45202

Chronic Pain Service
Department of Anesthesia
University Hospitals of Cleveland
2065 Adelbert Road
Cleveland, OH 44106

Pain Clinic
Rusk Rehabilitation Center
Columbus, OH 43216

Pain and Stress Treatment Center
Grant Hospital
Columbus, OH 43216

Elyria Acupuncture and Biofeedback Clinic
100 East Broad Street, Suite 4
Elyria, OH 44035

Section of Neurological Surgery
Department of Neurosciences
Medical College of Ohio
P. O. Box 6190
Toledo, OH 43601

Mercy Hospital
2200 Jefferson Avenue
Toledo, OH 43601

Pain Clinic
St. Elizabeth Medical Center
Youngstown, OH 44501

Youngstown Osteopathic Hospital
Box 1258
Youngstown, OH 44501

Oklahoma
University of Oklahoma
University Hospital and Clinics
Veterans Administration Hospital
Oklahoma City, OK 73100

Doctors' Medical Center
2325 South Harvard
Tulsa, OK 74101

Oregon
Sacred Heart Hospital
1200 Alder Street
Eugene, OR 97401

South Oregon Pain Clinic
Providence Hospital
Medford, OR 97501

Acupuncture Pain Control Center
7227 S. W. Terwilliger
Portland, OR 97208

Northwest Pain Center
Woodland Park Hospital
Portland, OR 97208

Pain Evaluation Clinic
1120 N. W. 20th
Good Samaritan Hospital
Portland, OR 97208

The Portland Pain Center
Emanuel Rehabilitation
Portland, OR 97208

Pennsylvania
Pain Clinic and Acupuncture
141 Salem Avenue
Carbondale, PA 18407

Low Back Pain Clinic
Crozer—Chester Medical Center
Upland
Chester, PA 19013

Willis C. Barnes, M.D.
Pain Clinic
115 Depot Street
Clarks Summit, PA 18411

Pain Clinic—Acupuncture
Delaware County Memorial Hospital
Drexel Hill, PA 19026

Du Bois Hospital
Du Bois, PA 15801

Polyclinic Hospital
Polyclinic Avenue
Harrisburg, PA 17105

Therapeutic and Diagnostic Pain Clinic of Conemaugh
Valley Memorial Hospital
1086 Franklin Street
Johnstown, PA 15909

Latrobe Nerve Block and Pain Studies Clinic
Latrobe Area Hospital
Latrobe, PA 15650

Allegheny Valley Hospital
1300 Carlisle Street
Natrona Heights, PA 15065

Misericordia Division
Mercy Catholic Medical Center
54th Street and Cedar Avenue
Philadelphia, PA 19139

Naval Regional Medical Center
Philadelphia, PA 19145

Pain Control Center of Temple University
Temple University Hospital
3401 North Broad Street
Philadelphia, PA 19104

Thomas Jefferson University Hospital
1025 Walnut Street
Philadelphia, PA 19104

University of Pennsylvania School
of Veterinary Medicine
North Bolton Center
Kennett Square
Philadelphia, PA 19104

Pain Control Center
University of Pittsburgh
Presbyterian University Hospital
Pittsburgh, PA 15219

Shadyside Hospital
5230 Centre Avenue
Pittsburgh, PA 15219

Veterans Administration Hospital
Pittsburgh, PA 15240

Guthrie Clinic, Ltd
Sayre, PA 18840

Rhode Island
Institute for Behavioral Medicine
Summit Medical Center
Providence, RI 02904

Rhode Island Hospital
Eddy Street
Providence, RI 02904

South Carolina
Medical University of South Carolina
Charleston, SC 29401

Richland Memorial Hospital
3301 Harden Street
Columbia, SC 29203

Tennessee
University of Tennessee Pain Clinic
66 North Pauline
Memphis, TN 38101

Texas
High Plains Baptist Hospital
Amarillo, TX 79107

Pain Evaluation and Treatment Center
University of Texas
Health Science Center
Dallas, TX 75221

Pain Relief Center
Division of Texas Neurological Institute
Medical City, Suite 109
7777 Forest Lane
Dallas, TX 75219

Pain Therapy Association
4000 Junius
Dallas, TX 75221

Presbyterian Hospital of Dallas
8210 Walnut Hill Lane, Suite 515
Dallas, TX 75219

Veterans Administration Hospital
4500 South Lancaster Road
Dallas, TX 75219

St. Mary's Hospital
404 8th Street
Galveston, TX 77550

Garland Pain Clinic
Memorial Hospital of Garland
Garland, TX 75040

Houston Pain Clinic
6608 Fannin
Suite 1417
Houston, TX 77002

Memorial City General Hospital
Houston, TX 77002

Texas Institute for Rehabilitation and Research
1333 Moursund Avenue
Texas Medical Center
Houston, TX 77002

University of Texas
Anesthesiology Pain Clinic
6400 West Cullen
Houston, TX 77002

University of Texas
Medical School at Houston
6400 West Cullen Street
Houston, TX 77002

Highland Hospital
4809 University Avenue
Suite 206
Lubbock, TX 79408

Pain Control Clinic
University of Texas
Health Science Center
San Antonio, TX 78228

Santa Rosa Baptist
Community Hospital
San Antonio, TX 78205

Wilford Hall Hospital
San Antonio, TX 78205

Utah
W. Lynn Richards, M.D.
480 South 400 East
Bountiful, UT 84010

University of Utah
College of Medicine
50 North Medical Drive
Salt Lake City, UT 84101

Virginia
University of Virginia Medical Center
Box 293
Charlottesville, VA 22903

The Memorial Hospital
Department of Anesthesia
Danville, VA 24541

National Capital Center for Craniofacial Pain
803 West Broad Street
Falls Church, VA 22046

Chippenham Hospital
7101 Jahnke Road
Richmond, VA 23219

Medical College of Virginia
Box 907
Richmond, VA 23219

McGuire Veterans Administration Hospital
Richmond, VA 23219

Washington
Pain Clinic
Harborview Medical Center
Seattle, WA 98101

Operant Program for Chronic Pain
Department of Rehabilitation Medicine
University Hospital
Seattle, WA 98105

School of Dental Medicine
Seattle, WA 98105

Seattle Veterans Administration Hospital Pain Clinic
Seattle, WA 98105

Swedish Hospital Medical Center
Seattle, WA 98101

University of Washington Hospital
University Hospital
Seattle, WA 98105

Virginia Mason Pain Clinic
Seattle, WA 98101

United General Hospital
Sedro Woolley, WA 98284

Sacred Heart Medical Center
West 101 8th Avenue
Spokane, WA 99210

Lakewood General Hospital
100th Street
Tacoma, WA 98402

Walla Walla General Hospital
1025 South Second Avenue
Walla Walla, WA 99362

West Virginia
Marshall University School of Medicine
Appalachian Regional Hospital
Veterans Hospital
Beckley, WV 25801

West Virginia University
Medical Center
Morgantown, WV 26505

H. J. Thomas Memorial Hospital
4605 MacCorkle Avenue, S.W.
South Charleston, WV 25303

Wisconsin
Trinity Memorial Hospital
5900 South Lake Drive
Cudahy, WI 53110

Pain and Health Rehabilitation Center
Route 2, Welsh Conlee
LaCrosse, WI 54601

Pain Management Unit
Rehabilitation Medicine
University of Wisconsin Hospitals
Madison, WI 53703

University of Wisconsin Center for Health Sciences
University of Wisconsin
Neurological and Rehabilitation Hospital
Madison, WI 53703

Medical College of Wisconsin
Milwaukee County Medical Complex
Milwaukee, WI 53202

St. Michael Hospital
2400 West Villard Avenue
Milwaukee, WI 53202

Veterans Administration Center
5000 West National Avenue
Milwaukee, WI 53202

Puerto Rico
San Juan Pain Clinic
Calle 16, No. 461. Ext. San Augustín
Rio Piedras, Puerto Rico 00928

FIVE
CARING FOR
THE ILL

Some personal crises transcend all consideration of age or level of development. One of these crises, which none of us wants to think about as happening to us or our loved ones, is illness or hospitalization. But these crises do come, so we all need to know something about caring for the ill.

Certain attitudes should be developed in order to be effective in visiting or caring for a sick person. First, the visit must be purposeful, so certain aims and goals for the visit should be determined before the visit is made. In other words, we should anticipate the patient's physical, mental, emotional, and spiritual needs, and how each of these relate to one another.

Second, we should be accepting of the patient and his situation of illness. We should not be judgmental, condemning, or vindictive. We must meet the patient where he is rather than where we are. Most important in this regard is the patient's right to privacy. We should not ask questions concerning anything about which the patient does not volunteer information.

Third, we should always maintain confidentiality. The patient should know that we will not tell anyone anything that he desires not to be public knowledge. Trust has some powerful healing antidotes in a time of despair.

Fourth, as a visitor, we should know our own strengths and weaknesses. When we know our limitations as well as our potential, we will be far more effective. Then we do not get involved in areas where we could possibly cause more harm or despair.

Fifth, an essential ingredient is empathy. *Sympathy* relates, "I feel sorry for you." *Empathy* says, "I am seeing the situation through your eyes and I care for you." Caring for a person and pitying a person are remarkably different things.

Sixth, a positive attitude of laughter is appropriate when used with discretion. Laughter is wholesome and stimulating to both patient and visitor. Smiles have helped where antibiotics have failed. But be sure that smiles and laughter are timely, for inappropriate laughter could cause more harm and damage.

BEING AN EFFECTIVE VISITOR

To be an effective and comforting visitor:

1. Knock on the door and receive permission to enter an ill person's room.

2. Walk in and talk softly as you approach the patient.

3. Identify yourself immediately if there is any question as to whether or not the patient will know you.

4. Give a warm appropriate handshake or embrace as a greeting if the patient is able to receive it.

5. Smile and have a pleasant facial expression.

6. Make the visit brief, assuring the patient that you will visit at length when he is feeling better. And if you promise to do so, do it. But be sensitive. You should be able to tell if the patient truly desires for you to stay longer. Yet, do not tire out the patient.

7. Keep in mind that the patient's condition is personal, so consider his rights of confidentiality.

8. Keep your personal problems to yourself. Be positive and affirming rather than negative.

The ill person needs to be free from negative influences so that all his energy can be used to maintain health. The goal of the care-giver is to provide relief from negative symptoms so patient and family can be comfortable and alert. The patient as well as the family thrive best when their own life-style and philosophy are respected and maintained.

Rarely can one person fully meet all the needs of an ill person. Care usually requires collaboration of many disciplines and persons working as a health-care team. Overall caring involves receiving as well as giving. This principle will be realized as people who care provide for one another through mutual support.

TEN COMMANDMENTS FOR CARING

At some point in all of our lives, we will be in the position of caring for an ill person. Many people are uncomfortable when they are called upon to make a hospital visit or to try to help people who have a life-threatening disease. Dr. Paul Johnson has related his "ten commandments"[1] for caring.

1. *Always tell the truth.* Yet, we do not have to tell *all* the truth at once. Speak the truth with love and sensitivity. Never belittle the problem or minimize its seriousness for the sake of false reassurance. Integrity in this area will help to build a trust relationship in which ministry can take place.

2. *Never set times.* No one can tell how much time a person has to live. Many so-called "hopeless" cases have had a reversal and have recovered. No doctor can speak with certainty about the termination of life.

3. *Listen with sensitivity.* It is important to find out what the ill person wants to talk about and let him guide the conversation. It is also important to admit "I

don't know" to questions for which we don't have answers rather than to provide misinformation.

4. *Respond to needs.* It is important to listen for clues to the concerns that trouble the ill person. Be alert to the ill person's economic, psychological, family, and other needs, and help when needs are revealed.

5. *Never allow the person to feel abandoned.* Often great care is taken medically to meet physical needs while emotional needs may be ignored. Calls, cards, flowers, and visits are all important and meaningful. It is particularly important that one never make a promise that he can't keep.

6. *Make yourself available.* It is important to be available at the ill person's request. Generally, long visits are not helpful, nor are more than two visitors at a time. Short frequent visits are the most meaningful.

7. *Do not give medical advice.* All too often well-meaning but ill-advised comments are made by visitors. Leave the medical advice and treatment to the professionals. If the person is unhappy or uncertain about his care, other doctors can and will be called for consultation.

8. *If necessary, protect the person from himself.* At times ill persons will attempt to treat themselves without telling their doctor, or will fail to take medication. The doctor needs to know about all attempts at self-treatment in case they might affect the treatment that has been prescribed.

9. *Always hold out hope.* However dark the situation, there is always something to be thankful for and cause for meaningful spiritual hope. Yet, be realistic in how you hold out hope to an ill person.

10. *Provide spiritual support.* Relationship with God is vital for a living or dying person. Be open and honest about your faith. Avoid heavy theological discussions and demands. But do share the simplicity of God's love and presence in simple affirmation and prayer.

PART II
DEATH AND DYING

SIX
WHY DEATH HAPPENS

When a loved one dies, most people go through a period of questioning the existence of God and sometimes even the purpose of their own existence. To better understand life and death, we must blend reason and faith. It is not rude or irreverent to question God if the question is done in faith as part of an honest search for truth and meaning. Questioning God is wrong, though, if it becomes a challenge to God, in unbelief and rebellion.

The wrong kind of why usually does not call for an answer but for an argument. We demand to know the ultimate why. In our grief we want answers and comfort.

God, I believe, has a grand scheme of things in design, although I can't always figure out all the primary reasons for things happening as they do. God is sovereign in the design of life and death. The why of an honest search for answers is not the same as the rebellious, belligerent why asked with a clenched fist.

The right kind of questioning can bring about some comfort for human understanding. Appropriate questioning also reveals some of the secondary purposes. Within God's love and sovereignty interact four major secondary variables to which man is subjected because of the direct or indirect result of the fall of man. These secondary variables are the laws of nature, human imperfection, community living, and divine impartiality.[1]

1. *The laws of nature.* God set certain natural, indiscriminating, natural laws into motion. If we accept the assets of nature, such as beauty, health, and wealth, then we must also accept the liabilities of nature such as disease, tornadoes, floods, and earthquakes. Disease is one of the laws of nature. There are no simple answers for why some people contract diseases and others never seem to be sick. If we blame God, then we have an inadequate theology or concept of who he is and how he works.

The material environment God has provided finds its stability in the fact that it is law-abiding. The rain may aid one set of human purposes and harm another. It may seem that the world and the environment are cruel and hopeless, but in them both there is stability and balance.

God does not always heal diseased physical bodies. A Christian doctor told me that he prayed for healing, "if it is God's will." He never tells patients that they will be physically healed if they have enough faith. People who say that God always heals if a person only has enough faith are strangely inconsistent. These same ones often wear false teeth, glasses, and other artificial aids. In the Bible there is a principle which could be called the "economy of the miraculous." God doesn't usually work a miracle when there is a normal way available, nor does he always intervene when the case is medically hopeless.

2. *Human imperfection.* Man is a frail framework. He cannot always see what is ultimately best or right. He makes decisions and must live with their consequences whether good or bad. Many times people blame God for accidents or mistakes when the real reasons for them are human imperfection.

A plane crash in a storm may point out human imperfection in man's decision-making processes. The pilot or his superiors saw the storm. They could have gone around it or over it or turned back. But they decided that it would be all right to go through it. The raging storm was worse than they had anticipated and something dreadful happened. No one knows for sure. The tragic plane crash was a result of human imperfection in reasoning concerning what to do about the approaching storm.

Accidents are usually a result of someone's imperfect reasoning. The automobile accident could have been avoided if the drivers had been responsible and considerate of each other. If automobiles go fast enough to provide needed transportation, they will also go fast enough to destroy lives.

Disease may result from imperfect reasoning. The food is delicious so we gorge ourselves. Perhaps some of the foods we eat contain elements that react against our bodies and cause certain unexplainable diseases. We know that certain processed food products may not be healthful, yet we continue to eat them.

Perhaps we did not do the right thing at the right time in order to avoid becoming ill. We may not have sought proper medical attention at the proper time. It is often our imperfect reasoning powers that get us into problems. Most of the time we are asking why God does not do something to help us in these matters, and he is probably expecting us to do more with our knowledge and abilities.

3. *Community living.* We do not live to ourselves in this world. As the world population grows, we realize that what one person does has an effect on others. When one person gets the flu, usually many other people get it. Epidemics take their toll.

Often when one person does something out of order some bystanders are affected. In other words, because we live and function in groups of people, sometimes one person may be responsible for another person's death.

A young man climbed to the top of the tower of the University of Texas campus, pulled out a gun, and began shooting students in all directions. Then the man shot himself. Because he lived in a community, Charles Whitman, in the University of Texas tower, not only hurt himself with a gun but also hurt twenty-one other people. If Whitman had been on a desert island, it would have been a different story. But he was in a community of people and his actions hurt many innocent people.

In community living, tragedies may result if people are not responsible and considerate of each other. In our contemporary society the misuse of alcohol and drugs has taken an overwhelming toll in harming people. Many innocent people have been harmed by another person who is under the influence of drugs.

So, even though it seems senseless, many times the actions of others bring harm or death to innocent by-standers.

4. *Divine impartiality.* "Good" comes to good people and bad people. "Bad" comes to good people and bad people. It rains on the just and the unjust. Think, for example, of the two houses and foundations of sand and rock mentioned in Matthew (7:24-27). The storms, rain, and wind came to both houses. They did not just come to the house on the sand. The house on the rock stood, but it did go through the storm. I sometimes think that although it stood, the house probably had to be reshingled or replastered in spots. But it did stand. If the foundation of a person's life is God's Word, he will be standing during and after the storm.

When I was in deep sorrow, going through a storm, doubts flooded my mind. At a major crisis point, I made the following statement of commitment:

> As I walk the way of inquiry that has produced doubt, uncertainty, and rank skepticism, I'm not afraid to en-

trust an unknown immediate future to my known God.

So many things have happened that could make my actions be based on superstition, but I'm not afraid to entrust an unknown immediate future to my known God.

I've endeavored in many seemingly worthwhile activities that have produced few visible affirmative results, but I'm not afraid to entrust an unknown immediate future to my known God.

When I ask why, I realize that God wants me to know: "My little child, if you could see it the way I see it, you would not worry. You would know that I am taking care of you in a very special way." I'm not afraid to entrust an unknown immediate future to my known God.

Perhaps, due to some of the things we have mentioned, some of us have been victims of some of these natural, indiscriminating laws of nature, human imperfection, community living, or what seems to be divine impartiality. I have felt that way many times.

But later on, I became aware that some of the grumbling I had done about my situation and my unanswered questions was not against the situation—it was against God!

In such situations, I wonder if God isn't thinking: "I must be faithful to man. He is trusting himself, his friends, his family, and society rather than trusting me. I must send him the circumstances that will help him to choose to trust in me."

To be sensible in these difficult circumstances is to be dependent on God. In order to understand and adjust, a Christian, through God's Word, must learn to think the way God thinks. We must learn to respond, "Thank you, Lord, that you are in charge" (1 Thessalonians 5:18).

God is sovereign. The devil could not tempt man until God permitted him to do so. In the Book of Job, chapters 38 to 40, Job asked the question, "Why did all the sorrow and grief come to me?" He tried to tell God that there was a better way to do things. Job thought he was wise. Then Job was asked some questions, which proved God's providence and sovereignty. When Job realized who God was and when he learned more about God's plans, he responded, "I don't know everything. How could I ever find the answers? I lay my hand upon my mouth in silence. I have said too much already."

Some of the answers to our whys, to our unanswerable questions, have already been revealed when God revealed himself to us in his Word. More answers come when he shows us more of who we are and what lies in our subconscious minds. Because he trusts himself to us, he lets the dark storms come. But all the time he continues to work. Rather than questioning God, we must stop and thank him for life itself, and for the life and work of the loved one we have lost.

SEVEN
THE DYING
PROCESS

Few people have little or no advance notice of their approaching death. Many people meet immediate death through accidents, or they never regain consciousness after an accident. Some lapse into coma from what was thought to have been a minor health problem. Some die of sudden illnesses, such as heart attacks or strokes. Others are the victims of homicide.

Most people, however, die of illnesses that prolong the dying process. Usually such deaths occur after a long illness, and the dying person is confined at home or in a hospital or some other institution.

Intellectually, we realize that we began the process of dying at the moment of birth. Yet, talk about death is often taboo in our society. We seem to be too busy living to think about dying. Realistically, my process of dying begins when I learn that I am dying. For you, my process of dying begins when you learn that I am going to die.

The concepts of dying and death are very closely associated. It is hard to think about one without the other. Yet, there are some important differences in the way we should think about them. Dying refers to the process of coming to an end of life, while death refers to the event ending physical life on earth.

The process of dying is not a popular subject for discussion. Traditionally doctors have not paid much attention to it. Their greatest aim is to preserve life. Once preserving life is no longer possible, they tend to lose interest and move on to patients they believe they can help. Until recently the medical world reacted to death as if the subject were adequately covered in the childhood skip-rope jingle:

> Doctor, Doctor, will I die?
> Yes, my child, and so will I.

Attitudes toward dying and attitudes toward death differ widely. The fear of the process of dying seems to be universal. As one of my colleagues put it, "I'm not afraid of death—it's the dying that concerns me." Our fear of dying stems from the motive of self-preservation and of wanting always to be in control.

The fear of death, however, is not universal. Some people regard death with friendly acquiescence, with fond anticipation, and even fanatical hope. On the other hand, the fear of the process of dying stems from anxieties about being left alone in social isolation in the dying process. Most people want to have friends and family close during the dying time. The rare exception would be the person who chooses to go into voluntary exile.

Since the early 1970s, the death and dying movement in America has been concerned with the "proper" process of dying. This interest has come mostly from religious workers and from health-care professionals other than physicians. This movement has given rise to the growth of death counseling, grief counseling, and the hospice movement. It began among hospital staff people who were bearing the burden of caring for people going

94

through lingering deaths from chronic illnesses. Such people were putting a great strain on the hospital workers as well as the families of the dying.

It is not enough to focus just on the desires, needs, hopes, and fears of the dying person because his oncoming death also affects the living. Each person, whether dying or living, reacts to the imminence of death in his or her own way. Each one has ideas of how and under what conditions the person should die. These divergent views may lead to tension and conflict, but the wishes of the dying should be respected as much as possible.

For the person who is dying, the dying process may seem to be lonely, but the experience is shared by everyone concerned. Each person's actions and reactions have an influence on all the others. The process of dying cannot be successfully understood unless one focuses on both the living and the dying. In addition to the concerns for the dying person, attention must be given to the needs, rights, and expectations of the ones who are taking care of the dying person.

Telling someone that he is dying does not assure his understanding or acceptance. Values and attitudes are not the same for all people. We are all affected differently by customs and our background. Ethnic barriers and social class boundaries are difficult to understand and cross.

A person may learn he is dying from any number of sources. Some learn it directly from the medical professionals or from family members. Medical sociologists were the first to describe the way a person may become aware of oncoming death. The four general states or contexts are:

1. *Closed awareness.* In this context, others know that the patient has a terminal illness but the patient does not.

2. *Suspected awareness.* In this situation, the patient suspects that he may die, but he does not know for sure.

3. *Pretense awareness.* In this context, both the patient and others know that the patient is dying, yet everyone agrees to act as if this were not the case.

4. *Open awareness.* In this situation, both the patient and others know that the patient is dying.

Whether or not a person realizes that he is approaching the process of dying, there are specific decisions that should be made and tasks that should be performed. First, the person has to make several medical decisions, whether to accept or deny treatment and perhaps to determine the type of treatment.

Second, certain priorities must be set based on time, energies, and resources remaining. The dying person must be encouraged to be realistic in his expectations.

Third, the dying person must complete his unfinished business. He needs to express his personal desires, love, and appreciation as professional and personal decisions are being made.

Fourth, the dying person may need to make some arrangements for his family and personal affairs, matters that will concern his family after his death. Included in these arrangements are a legal will, a living will, insurance, funeral, and burial plans.

Fifth, the dying person must work with the task of coping with losses here on earth. These may include physical, emotional, mental, and social relationships.

Sixth, the person must deal with the physical mysteries of the process of dying. Anya Foos-Graber[1] has presented some new insights to the medical world in the process of dying. In her book entitled *Deathing*, she proposes a modern craft of dying—a right and conscious way of dying—which she calls "deathing." Usually when people die they are unprepared, uninformed, and frightened, especially if they are alone. She offers helpful hints to free up dying people so they can use the transition as a peak moment in the culmination of life on earth. This method teaches people ahead of time how to practice sensory perception, relaxation, and breathing. At the moment of death, the person will be awake, aware, responsible, and joyful. Preparation for deathing made beforehand can insure that the dying person will be ready—not unaware and helpless—at the final moment on earth.

Observing the process of a person dying is extremely difficult for the loved ones. Contrary to popular misconception, a person does not usually just stop breathing immediately. It is often a slow, lingering, unwinding process. This is a common phenomenon on a deathbed when the dying person's respiration becomes erratic. The medical term is Cheyne-Stokes[2] breathing patterns of dying.

The respiration cycle begins with slow, shallow breaths that gradually increase to abnormal depth and rapidity. Respiration subsides as breathing slows and becomes shallower, climaxing in a 10- to 20-second period without respiration before the cycle is repeated. Each cyclic episode may last from 45 seconds to 3 to 5 minutes.

The family will think that the person has stopped breathing, and in a few seconds or minutes later the person will take another breath. This is most traumatic for families to go through because they do not know when the person is totally dead. The emotional experience of the final few moments may be devastating.

Seventh, the dying person must deal with his oncoming encounter with the spiritual mysteries of death. In his classic book entitled Angels,[3] Billy Graham presents the scriptural concept of angels attending the Christian during the process of dying. The Bible teaches that death releases the Christian from this present world so that angels may transport believers to their heavenly inheritance. The Christian will actually be taken by angels into the presence of God.

Those who have made peace with God will be able to

say with D. L. Moody, "Some day you will read in the papers that D. L. Moody is dead. Don't you believe a word of it. At that moment I shall be more alive than I am now. . . . That which is born of flesh may die. That which is born of the Spirit will live forever."

Dying people are usually not totally conscious since they are often given drugs to take care of pain. Because of this, we do not hear about as many experiences of angels coming to carry the dying believer into the presence of the Lord. Most people, very naturally, fear the thought of dying and death, and no person is truly ready to die until he has learned to live. Billy Graham said, "You can put your confidence in Jesus because He died for you, and in that last moment—the greatest crisis of all—He will have His angels gather you in their arms to carry you gloriously, wonderfully into heaven."

The dying person has specific needs as he goes through certain stages in the process of dying. In the following chapter, we will discuss some of them.

EIGHT
NEEDS AND STAGES

One afternoon, during the death and dying class at the university, we were discussing the needs of a dying person. As the class discussion grew deeper, a student remarked: "People need people. Sick people need people. Dying people *really* need people!"

Once a person is labeled as dying, many people tend to treat him as a nonperson. Most people do not understand the needs and stages involved in a person's dying. Talcott Parsons, a well-known sociologist, has revealed some of the needs and expectations of a dying person:

1. The sick and dying person is expected to avoid any situation or behaviors that will make the terminal condition worse.

2. The dying person is expected to accept the personal and professional help that is needed as the condition intensifies.

3. The dying person is expected to desire to get better and want to live, or to release the desire to get better because death is inevitable.

4. The dying person is expected to realize that his needs are beyond the help of medical science. At this time, the patient's objective is to be as comfortable as possible in the completion of the process of dying.

A HIERARCHY OF NEEDS

Psychologist Abraham Maslow classified a system of human needs in terms of a hierarchy, a system adaptable also for the dying person.

1. *Physiological needs.* The dying as well as the living have the basic human needs for air, water, food, and physical comfort. When illness diminishes physical strength, there is a change in the way basic needs have to be met. Many times the diet has to be changed because it is no longer possible to eat some foods. When breathing becomes more difficult, artificial respiration may be required. Perhaps the greatest physical need is that of dealing with pain.

The physical conditions that cause the most problems are an increase in loss of strength and attractiveness, loss of bowel and urinary control, choking, and pain. Health-care consumers need to know about physical care that is available to the terminally ill.

2. *Safety and security needs.* The dying person has more need to feel safe and secure than ever before. First, he feels insecure due to his lack of trust in his medical care. When the patient realizes that medical help is not working, then he tends to become insecure and distrustful of health-care professionals. The patient feels insecure also when he suspects that he does not know all the truth. There is a great need to maintain some feelings of control over one's life. For most people, when the body becomes ill, the total self is sick. Insecurity comes also when the terminally ill person feels that he is not getting his personal wishes met.

3. *Love and belonging needs.* The dying person's longing for affection often intensifies. It is not surprising that psychological needs at such a time are perhaps at their peak. The job of caring for an ill person ranges from encouraging him when his emotions are low to helping to fill the empty hours with something satisfying.

One of the greatest emotional problems for the dying

person is loneliness. People who are sick or dying want social interaction, but when their energy decreases they may withdraw by sleeping or becoming apathetic. Socializing may be wanted at times and not desired at other times, so caring for such people demands flexibility.

Psychologically, people are never too sick to need love, yet they are not always able to respond adequately to those expressing such love and care. Many times the terminally ill feel guilty for being sick, feelings that come from not wanting to be a burden or to cause trouble for those who are caring for them. Even though a person may not be able to express love to others, caring people must always continue to show love to them.

4. *Self-esteem needs.* Everyone has the need to "be somebody." Society dictates that "I am somebody" and "I am good" when I have accomplished something good. Since the dying process incapacitates the dying person, he feels helpless and dependent. Self-esteem is the overall feeling of value, dignity, and worth. Chronic illness produces the negative feelings of worthlessness, badness, and dependence.

Anything that wounds a person physically, psychologically, and socially also tests him spiritually. Serious illness robs a person of feelings of worth and deprives him of good feelings about himself. The dying person needs to be as involved as possible in his situation and with people who love him so that he will not feel nonproductive. Quite often, when a dying person feels he is of no worth, he complicates everything for himself and the people taking care of him.

5. *Self-actualization needs.* Everyone has the needs of personal growth and fulfillment. As the needs of a lower hierarchy are not satisfied, so also the higher needs are deeply frustrated. The dying person's self-actualization needs are intensified in several areas. These include his

unfulfilled dreams and his unfinished business. So many personally important things will not happen as he intended. Fulfillment needs demand that the chronically ill person find meaning in his life and death. One of the most fulfilling things the dying can do is to seek reconciliation within himself, with others, as well as with God.

It is difficult to provide care for a dying person who has so many different kinds of needs. Illness that disrupts living brings on needs on all different levels, from physical to spiritual. We do not simply start with the need lowest in the hierarchy and move up to another need only after the first has been met. Instead, we are faced with the enormous challenge of meeting physiological and self-esteem needs all at one time. If the patient does not feel good about himself, he will probably not participate in his physical and emotional care. Although we should not offer false hopes about his recovery, we can meet many needs that will gradually help to restore some of the patient's self-esteem.

Those who are taking care of the patient also have needs. They feel the need to be with the dying person and to be helpful. Being informed of conditions and impending death is a deep need for those who are taking care. They also need to feel the support and comfort from other family members as well as from the health professionals. Perhaps one of their greatest needs is to be able to ventilate their emotions and desires to someone who cares for them.

STAGES OF GRIEF

In addition to understanding the dying person's emotional needs, it is helpful to understand that dying people go through several rational and emotional stages in their process of dying. Elizabeth Kubler-Ross has described the stages through which the dying person goes.

Her book entitled *On Death and Dying*[1] has become a primary resource book for professionals and lay people working in the field of death and dying. Since most people who work in this area use Dr. Kubler-Ross's outline, it might be appropriate to look at these stages in the order in which they often come:

1. *Denial and isolation.* When a person receives the first diagnosis that he has a terminal illness, his first reaction is one of disbelief or denial. He usually says things such as, "Oh, no! This cannot be true!" or "There must be a mistake!" The person doesn't believe the medical reports and insists on repeat examinations. Often he begins to shop around for another doctor and another medical opinion. Denial is a temporary defense mechanism. It serves as a necessary buffer, a delaying mechanism against the overwhelming anxiety until the person can deal with the news.

During the time of denial, there is an intense feeling of isolation from loved ones, friends, and from the real world. Those giving care must wait through this first phase and let the person know that they are available and willing to listen when they desire to talk. If a dying person denies his illness for a prolonged time, even in spite of advancing symptoms, those who must care for him should give compassion and support as death comes closer. Extensive denial is unhealthy because it hinders the dying person's preparations to face the inevitable separation and grief. Yet, some people maintain their denial to the end. Denial is usually interrupted by the next stage, anger.

2. *Anger.* As anger rises, the patient goes through periods of rage, envy, and resentment. This second phase begins when the reality of the prognosis is established. The feelings of anger are usually displaced onto things or people. One might hear him say things like, "The doctor is no good," or "This hospital is terrible," "Nurses are neglectful," or "Nobody cares." The family and

health-care professionals usually bear the brunt of all this anger, but it can include ministers, and even God. No one, it seems, can do anything right to please him. The dying person becomes angry with all those who go on living.

Many questions arise in the midst of a person's anger. The major question is a belligerent "Why me?" This stage is very difficult to handle by medical professionals and the family. The dying person is not really angry at other people. He is really angry at death and the fact of his dying. Anger may not only be present in the beginning of awareness of dying. It can continue as long as the person has made no satisfactory resolution to death.

Anger has to be expressed and for the dying person it will eventually pass. It must not be taken personally. A calm approach is needed to help to lower anger and anxiety.

3. *Bargaining*. The third stage is bargaining, either conscious or unconscious, direct or indirect behavior expressed to others. The dying person tries to enter into some kind of agreement which may postpone death. Bargaining usually consists of promises with God, doctors, and family.

The dying patient says to God, "If you will let me live, then I will serve you." "If you heal me, I will read the Bible." He says to the doctors, "I will be a good patient if you will help me to get well. Promise me that I have another year to live." To the family, he says, "I will do (this or that) if you will help me to live. When I get well, I will _____."

It is important during this time to note in the dying person any underlying feelings of guilt or regrets about his life. We should listen to those expressions of regret and grief. During this time we can help him to become more realistic in his feelings.

As Dr. Kubler-Ross shows, a patient cannot keep the bargaining promises. He is like a little child who promises, "I will be good forever." Needless to say, the child gets into trouble the very next day.

4. *Depression.* When the patient realizes that bargaining won't help to bring health, the patient usually goes into a time of depression. During this time, dying people grieve over the loss of body image, their role in life, their relationships, and financial losses. Then they begin the grief of separating from life itself.

There are two major types of depression. Reactive depression is the sudden response to a great number of problems that a patient faces. There is first the shock of everything coming at once. Then there is preparatory depression, the normal grief the patient has to go through in order to prepare for separation from this world. The first reaction other people have to someone's depression is to try to cheer him up. This may meet the needs of the caring person, but not of the dying. At this point, the patient is not denying his approaching death, but is trying to "put it all together" and find personal meaning. This usually brings about the fifth stage of the grief process.

5. *Acceptance.* The dying person usually comes to this stage if given enough time and help. Unless there is an unexpected sudden death, all the stages may be completed. During this final stage, a patient may tend to separate himself from all of his relationships. He is, during this time, making his own preparations for death.

Acceptance is not necessarily defined as a happy stage. The patient does not say, "Great. I'm going to die." Instead, there may be very little emotion expressed, since this last stage is almost void of emotional feeling. Communication becomes more nonverbal than verbal. Acceptance takes the form of resignation and the patient seems ready to die with dignity. It has been best described by Stewart Alsop: "A dying person needs to die like a sleepy person needs to sleep."

With acceptance, the cycle of stages in the process of

dying is completed. Yet, the process of dying is too complicated to put such simplistic labels on a cycle. Not every dying person, for example, will experience all of these stages or in the order presented here. Yet, these five stages are usually the natural, normal progression in the life of a dying person.

When it has become clear to a person that he is dying and that death is inevitable, two major issues need to be faced. First, the dying person needs to receive permission, from the significant people he will leave behind, to pass away. A dying person should not be made to feel, by his loved ones, that his death is so unacceptable that it will take away all meaning and purpose from their lives. The dying person needs to know that life will somehow go on for the ones he leaves behind.

Second, the dying person needs to voluntarily release every person and possession that is significant to him. It is always better to have the feeling of surrendering gracefully those things we know we cannot keep rather than maintain the attitude that they are being snatched away from us.

HOSPICE CARE

The actual physical place where a terminally ill patient receives care and treatment and where he will actually die often has great significance for the patient and his family. Terminally ill people today usually die in a hospital. A few people, however, have chosen to die in their own homes. An increasing number are choosing to die under hospice care.

Hospice care is an approach to death designed to insure that the person dies comfortably, free from pain, and in an understanding support community of health professionals, other dying patients, and family members. Hospice care is sometimes provided by teams that come to the patient's home. Hospices are sometimes a professional medical "halfway house" for the dying, who choose not to die in a hospital nor at home.

The staff of approved hospices are clinically competent, ethically sound, psychologically helpful, and spiritually beneficial. The following is a list of hospice organization members in the United States.

Alabama
Villa Mercy, Inc.
P. O. Box 1096
101 Villa Drive
Daphne, AL 36526

Arizona
Hospice of the Valley
214 East Willette Street
Phoenix, AZ 85004

Hillhaven Hospice
5504 East Pima Street
Tucson, AZ 85712

Arkansas
N. W. Arkansas Hospice Association
P. O. Box 817
Fayetteville, AR 72701

Hospice of Jonesboro
Route 2, Box 182
Jonesboro, AR 72401

Hospice of the Ozarks
808 Church Street
Mountain Home, AR 72653

California
Hospice of Santa Cruz
330 Doris Avenue
Aptos, CA 95003

Hospice of Los Angeles
510 Doheny Road
Beverly Hills, CA 92410

Hospice at Parkwood
Parkwood Community Hospital
7011 Shoup Avenue
Canoga Park, CA 91304

Hospice of Monterey Peninsula
P. O. Box 7236
Carmel, CA 93921

El Cajon Valley Hospice Unit
1688 East Main Street
El Cajon, CA 92021

The Elizabeth Hospice
P. O. Box 891
Escondido, CA 92025

Hospice of Humbolt, Inc.
730 Harris Street
Eureka, CA 95501

Hospice of Fresno
St. Agnes Medical Center
1303 East Herndon Avenue
Fresno, CA 93710

Hospice of Granada Hills
Granada Hills Community Hospital
10445 Balboa Boulevard
Granada Hills, CA 91344

Kaiser Hayward Hospice
27400 Hesperian Boulevard
Hayward, CA 94545

Hospice of Orange County, Inc.
P. O. Box 2809
Laguna Hills, CA 92653

V.A. Wadsworth Medical Center
Wilshire and Sawtelle Boulevards
Los Angeles, CA 90073

V.N.A. Association of Los Angeles, Inc.
2538 West 8th Street
Los Angeles, CA 90073

Kaiser-Permanente Hospice Program
South Hoxie Avenue
Norwalk, CA 90650

Mercy General Hospital
4001 J Street
Sacramento, CA 95819

Bay Area Hospice Association
Hospice of San Francisco
14th Avenue and Lake Street
San Francisco, CA 94118

Vesper Hospice
311 MacArthur Boulevard
San Leandro, CA 74577

Hospice of Marin
77 Mark Drive, Suite 6
San Rafael, CA 94903

Hospice of Santa Barbara City
330 East Carrillo Street
Santa Barbara, CA 93101

Home Hospice of Sonoma County
P. O. Box 11546
Santa Rosa, CA 95406

Sonoma Valley Hospital District
P. O. Box 600
347 Andrieux Street
Sonoma, CA 95476

Hospice of the Conejo
1000 East Thousand Oaks Boulevard
Suite 224-D
Thousand Oaks, CA 91360

Hospice Care/Hospital Home Care
23228 Hawthorne Boulevard
Torrance, CA 90505

Hospice of Tulare County, Inc.
P. O. Box 781
Tulare, CA 93275

National In-Home Health Service
6850 Van Nuys Boulevard
Van Nuys, CA 91405

Hospice of Contra Costa
120 La Casa Via
Walnut Creek, CA 94596

Colorado
Boulder County Hospice
2118 14th Street
Boulder, CO 80302

Hospice of Metro Denver, Inc.
1719 East 19th Avenue
Room 256
Denver, CO 80218

Hospice, Inc., of Larimer County
P. O. Box 957
Fort Collins, CO 80522

Grand River Hospital District
701 East 5th Street
Rifle, CO 81650

Connecticut
Connecticut Hospice, Inc.
765 Prospect Street
New Haven, CT 06511

District of Columbia
The Washington Home
3720 Upton Street, N.W.
Washington, DC 20016

Washington Hospice Society
1828 L Street, N.W., Suite 505
Washington, DC 20036

Florida
Elizabeth Kubler-Ross Hospice
P. O. Box 6311
Clearwater, FL 33518

Halifax Hospital Medical Center
Clyde Morris Boulevard
Daytona Beach, FL 32015

Hospice of South Florida, Inc.
50 East Las Olas Boulevard
Ft. Lauderdale, FL 33301

Hospice of Broward, Inc.
3700 Washington Street, Suite 208
Hollywood, FL 33021

Methodist Hospital-Hospice
580 West 8th Street
Jacksonville, FL 32250

Hospice of Miami
127 N. E. 4th Street
Miami, FL 33132

Hospice of Orlando, Inc.
P. O. 8581
Orlando, FL 32806

Gold Coast Home Health Service
4699 North Federal Highway
Pompano Beach, FL 33064

Hospice of St. Francis, Inc.
P. O. Box 5563
Titusville, FL 32780

Hospice of Palm Beach County
P. O. Box 6562
West Palm Beach, FL 33405

Georgia
Hospice Atlanta, Inc.
P. O. Box 8376
Atlanta, GA 30306

Hawaii
St. Francis Hospital
2230 Liliha Street
Honolulu, HI 96817

Illinois
Horizon Hospice, Inc.
2430 North Lakeview
Chicago, IL 60614

Hospice of Madison County
2120 Madison Avenue
Granite City, IL 62040

Highland Park Hospital Hospice
718 Glenview Road
Highland Park, IL 60035

Evangelical Hospital Association
1415 West 22nd Street
Oak Brook, IL 60521

Indiana
Parkview Memorial Hospital
2200 Randalia Drive
Fort Wayne, IN 46805

Methodist Hospital of Indiana
1604 Capitol Avenue
Indianapolis, IN 46202

Hospice of Southern Indiana
134 East Main Street
New Albany, IN 47150

Iowa
Hospice of Central Iowa, Inc.
810 Walnut Street
Des Moines, IA 50309

Kentucky
E. McDowell Community Hospice
915 South Limestone
Lexington, KY 40506

Hospice of Louisville
233 East Gray Street
Suite 204
Louisville, KY 40222

Maine
Hospice of Maine
32 Thomas Street
Portland, ME 04102

Maryland
Church Hospital Corporation
100 North Broadway
Baltimore, MD 21231

Massachusetts
Hospice of the North Shore, Inc.
P. O. Box U
Beverly Farms, MA 01915

Michigan
Hospice of Flint
806 West 6th Avenue
Flint, MI 48503

Hurley Medical Center
One Hurley Plaza
Flint, MI 48502

Minnesota
Riveredge Hospice
P. O. Box 313
Breckenridge, MN 56520

St. Luke's Hospital
915 East First Street
Duluth, MN 55805

Fairview-Southdale Hospital
6401 France Avenue South
Minneapolis, MN 55435

North Memorial Medical Center
3220 Lowry Avenue North
Minneapolis, MN 55422

Bethesda Lutheran Medical Center
559 Capitol Boulevard
St. Paul, MN 55103

Missouri

Hospice Care of Mid-America
1005 Grand, Room 743
Kansas City, MO 64106

Lutheran Medical Center
Continuing Care Unit
2639 Miami
St. Louis, MO 63118

St. Luke's Hospital Hospice
35 North Central Avenue
St. Louis, MO 63105

New Jersey

Riverside Hospice
Powerville Road
Boonton, NJ 07005

Overlook Hospital Hospice
Home Care Department
193 Morris Avenue
Summit, NJ 07901

New York

Hospice Buffalo, Inc.
2929 Main Street
Buffalo, NY 14214

Calvary Hospital
1740 Eastchester Road
New York, NY 10461

Columbia University Foundation of Thanatology
Hospice Program
730 Park Avenue
New York, NY 10021

St. Luke's Hospital Center Hospice
Amsterdam Avenue at 114th Street
New York, NY 10025

Hospice of Rockland, Inc.
Rockland County Health Center
Pomona, NY 10970

United Hospital Hospice
406 Boston Post Road
Port Chester, NY 10573

Mercy Hospital
1000 North Village Avenue
Rockville Center, NY 11570

North Carolina
Hospice of North Carolina
Box 312
Duke University Medical Center
Durham, NC 27710

Ohio
Hospice of Cincinnati, Inc.
P. O. Box 19221
Cincinnati, OH 45219

Hospice of Dayton, Inc.
One Wyoming Street, Suite 430
Dayton, OH 45409

Pennsylvania
The Bryn Mawr Hospital
Bryn Mawr Avenue
Bryn Mawr, PA 19010

A. Einstein Medical Center, N. D.
York and Tabor Roads
Philadelphia, PA 19141

Hospice Philadelphia, Inc.
1900 Spruce Street
Philadelphia, PA 19103

Presbyterian Medical Center
51 North 39th Street
Philadelphia, PA 19104

Hospital Program of Pennsylvania Hospital
8th and Spruce Streets
Philadelphia, PA 19107

Forbes Health System
500 Finley Street
Pittsburgh, PA 15206

Hospice of St. John
191 North Franklin Avenue
Wilkes-Barre, PA 18702

Valley Crest Nursing Center
Route 115
Plains Township
Wilkes-Barre, PA 18711

Rhode Island
Hospice Care of Rhode Island
157 A Waterman Street
Providence, RI 02906

Tennessee
Fort Sanders Hospice
Fort Sanders Presbyterian Hospital
1901 Clinch Avenue, S.W.
Knoxville, TN 37916

Texas
Girling and Associates Home
Health Service, Inc.
1404 North Loop
Austin, TX 78756

Home Health-Home Care, Inc.
904 28th Street
Orange, TX 77630

Southeast Texas Hospice
312 Pine Street
Orange, TX 77630

St. Benedict's Hospice
330 East Johnson
San Antonio, TX 78201

Virginia
Hospice of Northern Virginia, Inc.
P. O. Box 2590
Arlington, VA 22210

Fairfax Nursing Center
Hospice Program
10701 Main Street
Fairfax, VA 22030

Riverside Hospital
500 J. Clyde Morris Boulevard
Newport News, VA 23601

Roanoke Memorial Hospital
Belleview at Jefferson Street
Roanoke, VA 24014

Edmarc Hospital for Children, Inc.
P. O. Box 1684
Suffolk, VA 23434

Wisconsin
Bellin·Hospice
Bellin Hospital
Box 1700
744 South Webster
Green Bay, WI 54305

Milwaukee Hospice, Inc.
1022 North 9th Street
Milwaukee, WI 53233

Visiting Nurse Association
of Milwaukee
Home Health Services
1540 North Jefferson Street
Milwaukee, WI 53202

Rogers Memorial Hospital Hospice
34810 Pabst Road
Oconomowoc, WI 53066

Washington
Hospice of Seattle
819 Boylson
Seattle, WA 98104

Hospice Maranatha
1620 North Monroe
Spokane, WA 99201

Hospice of Tacoma
742 Market Street, Suite 201
Tacoma, WA 98402

NINE
DEFINITION
OF DEATH

Death is another one of the medical mysteries from which the general public has been excluded. A proper explanation of it has not been made a part of the journey of life. The medical world has described death from two different health perspectives. From the biomedical or mechanistic view, contemporary medicine has attained heights of curing potential never before realized. Dying, in this view, is the ultimate illness, which should be treated and controlled for as long as possible.

The other, the wholistic view, is that death is part of life, just the last stage of the growth process. Death is normal and a natural process, not something to be resisted at all cost by any means. From this viewpoint, the physician helps people to understand that there are fates far worse than death. He helps the patient make decisions about the time and circumstances of death. According to this view, death is a transition back to the presence of God.

A dying person should choose his view and make it known to his physician, family, and friends. Above all, each person should act upon his choice when the time comes.

Someone once spoke of death as the final boundary line situation that sums up the whole of life. He spoke also of the many ways in which death takes on a paradoxical nature. While it is inevitable and universal, something that cannot be taken lightly, it still cannot be considered a common everyday happening. Though widespread and certain for everyone to undergo, each death resists common treatment. Death always presents itself as an extraordinary event. Each death is unique, and no one can do our dying for us.

Man, unlike the animals, knows that he is someday going to die. Yet, the paradox remains. We know we are going to die and still there is great difficulty in believing it.

Medicine's present ability to prolong life signals a need for serious debate on the issue of when death occurs. The time has come for us to stop trying to hide from the highly complex questions. We must give attention to our most competent physicians, religious leaders, and politicians to give us an acceptable and legal definition of death.

The present definition of death poses problems to the contemporary medical world. In its simplest form, death is described two different ways. One is "heart-death," when the heart and respiration stops. The other is "brain-death," when the brain ceases to function but the rest of the body—heart, lungs, and other organs—continues to function.

The Harvard Medical School commissioned a task force on death and dying for the determination of brain death. The following criteria was presented and described:[1]

1. *Unreceptivity and unresponsivity.* There is a total unawareness to externally applied stimuli and inner need and complete unresponsiveness—our definition of irreversible coma. Even the most intensely painful stimuli evoke no vocal or other responses, not even a groan,

withdrawal of limb, or quickening of respiration.

2. *No movements or breathing.* Observation covering a period of at least one hour by physicians is adequate to satisfy the criteria of no spontaneous muscular movements or spontaneous respiration or response to stimuli such as pain, touch, sound, or light. After the patient is on a mechanical respirator for three minutes it is observed that there is no effort on the part of the subject to breathe spontaneously. (The respirator may be turned off for this time provided that at the start of the trial period the patient's carbon dioxide tension is within the normal range, and provided also that the patient has been breathing room air for at least ten minutes prior to the trial.)

3. *No reflexes.* Irreversible coma with abolition of central nervous system activity is evidenced in part by the absence of elicitable reflexes. The pupil will be fixed and dilated and will not respond to a direct source of bright light. Since the establishment of a fixed, dilated pupil is clear-cut in clinical practice, there should be no uncertainty as to its presence. Ocular movement (to head turning and to irrigation of the ears with ice water) and blinking are absent. There is no evidence of postural activity (decerebrate or other). Swallowing, yawning, vocalization are in abeyance. Corneal and pharyngeal reflexes are absent.

As a rule, the stretch tendon reflexes cannot be elicited; i.e., tapping the tendons of the biceps, triceps, and pronator muscles, quadriceps and gastronemius muscles with the reflex hammer elicits no contraction of the respective muscles. Plantar or noxious stimulation gives no response.

4. *Flat electroencephalogram.* Of great confirmatory value is the flat or isoelectric EEG. We must assume that the electrodes have been properly applied, that the apparatus is functioning normally, and that the personnel in charge is competent. We consider it prudent to have

one channel of the apparatus used for an electrocardiogram. This channel will monitor the ECG so that if it appears in the electroencephalographic leads because of high resistance it can be readily identified. It also establishes the presence of the active heart in the absence of EEG. We recommend that another channel be used for a noncephalic lead. This will pick up space-borne or vibration-borne artifacts and identify them. The simplest form of such a monitoring noncephalic electrode has two leads over the dorsum of the hand, preferably the right hand, so that ECG will be minimal or absent. Since one of the requirements of this state is that there be no muscle activity, these two dorsal hand electrodes will not be bothered by muscle artifact. [The article went on to describe in somewhat technical terms the range of settings for the apparatus.] . . . At least ten full minutes of recording are desirable, but twice that would be better.

It is also suggested that the gains at some point be opened to their full amplitude for a brief period (5 to 100 seconds) to see what is going on. Usually in an intensive care unit artifacts will dominate the picture, but these are readily identifiable. There shall be no electroencephalographic response to noise or to pinch.

All of the above tests shall be repeated at least twenty-four hours later with no change.

The validity of such data as indications of irreversible cerebral damage depends on the exclusion of two conditions: hypothermia (temperature below 90° F [32.2° C]) or central nervous system depressants such as barbiturates.

The criteria are clear and distinct; the medical exams are easily performed and interpreted by the doctors. These criteria do not require the attending physician to declare the patient "dead" but do substantiate medical proof for death. Therefore, it is still up to the physician and family to declare when a person is dead.

TEN
OVERCOMING THE
FEAR OF DEATH

One afternoon I was visiting with a young child who was dying. As I was leaving the hospital room, she asked me if we could pray together before I left. As I was getting ready to pray for her, she began:

> Lord,
> If I have to die,
> Let me die;
> But please,
> Take away the fear.

In dealing with the fear of death, we are confronted with the question of which is the cause and which is the effect. We fear what we do not understand. Avoidance of death and the anxiety we experience about it are interrelated. Our behavior changes during experiences that make us anxious or frightened. There are a variety of ways in which a person may express his fears and try to overcome them.

1. *Avoidance.* Directly or indirectly, people tend to avoid what they fear. Someone may respond to the funeral of a friend in ways that show he is trying to avoid death and the thoughts of death. Someone avoiding

death might say, "I am not going to the funeral because funerals make me very depressed." Another might say, "I do not want to talk about it." Such people seem to be saying that if they don't think or talk about death, they can successfully avoid it altogether.

2. *Changing life-styles.* Many Americans have recently made drastic changes in their health and eating habits as if by doing so they may postpone death. This new approach includes a new emphasis on food preparation, exercise, vitamins, and rest. People today are also eating less junk food, avoiding preservatives and additives, and eating more natural foods.

Some of them, when they learn what they ought to eat, find themselves in a dilemma since it is hard to know how to buy and prepare healthful foods. In trying to get back to better living habits, avoiding such things as smoking, alcohol, and drugs, they are, in many cases, demonstrating their unspoken fear of death and dying.

3. *Dreams and fantasies.* In our dreams and fantasies, we are letting down our psychological guard, allowing our true feelings and thoughts to surface in visual forms. Many of our nocturnal dreams as well as our daydreams are subconscious attempts to express and deal with our fears of death. For example, some people are obsessed with repressed feelings or fears of their own death. They may be plagued with dreams that leave them emotionally devastated. Some will fantasize their own funeral in order to work through their fears about death. People who hold unhealthy concepts about death and dying will reflect these fears and anxieties in their dreams.

4. *Challenging death.* Many people indirectly express their fears by constantly challenging death, and winning. Some challenge death through danger in their work and play. Such persons are sometimes called "daredevils." They seem to get a thrill out of daring death to take them. When they challenge death and

win, they feel superior to death. Usually such actions give a false idea that they can always win against death, that they will never die.

5. *Humor.* Some people resort to defensive humor to try to establish their superiority over death, by making it seem like some kind of a joke. After all, we have heard that we are greater than the things we can laugh about, so we try to conquer death and our fear of death by humor. As long as we are laughing, we do not have to think too much about it.

6. *Displacing fears.* A few people try to displace their fears of death through work or entertainment. To displace means "to take the place of" something else. A person may get so involved in his work and in being successful that in the long run it makes his fear of death seem small. Usually this type of person has a great amount of anxiety and gets depressed often.

7. *Becoming a professional.* In order to deal with fear, a person may become a professional or paraprofessional in an area related to his fear. A person who fears death may become a physician, nurse, counselor, minister, or teacher. When a person realizes that he has a fear of death, many times he chooses to conquer the fear by getting involved with death and dying on a professional level.

Everyone, regardless of age, has some general fears about death and dying. These fears are wrapped up in certain losses that they anticipate, such as loss of control, loss of self-confidence, loss of good health, loss of privacy and modesty, loss of productivity and self-fulfillment, and the loss of their plans for the future. When we consider the possibility of our own death, we feel specific concerns and fears according to our age and position in life. At different ages we fear different things that would result from our death. Some of these specific concerns, according to the decades of life,[1] might be:

Teens:
Not marrying
Not becoming a parent
Not having enough time to become a professional
Twenties:
Leaving family
How loved ones would cope with grief
Financial and emotional burdens on the family
Lack of significant accomplishment
Thirties:
Female:
Abandonment of children
Guilt feelings
Not living to see children grown
Male:
Financial security for family
End of productivity
Loss of control
Forties:
Welfare of spouse
Welfare of children
Financial security of survivors
Dread of separation
Fifties:
Welfare of family
Welfare of children
Welfare of grandchildren
Anxiety about extended suffering
Fear of the process of dying
Sixties, Seventies, and Eighties:
Welfare of families
Fear of being kept alive beyond hope of recovery
Fear of control of estate

We all have fears and anxieties about approaching the unknown, especially death. As we said earlier, there is usually a greater fear of the process of dying than of death itself. When a person has learned to adjust and cope in life, he will probably better respond to coping and adjusting to death. In other words, if a person has difficulty facing life he will have difficulty facing death.

A great deal of time has been given to the discussion of fears about death and dying. It is important to see that there are some profound ways of overcoming those fears. One semester, in my course at the university on death and dying, I asked, "What is the first step in overcoming fears about death?" After a moment of silence, one student suggested, "A successful and happy life begins with understanding that we will die."

Another student told about almost dying in an auto accident. He said, "There were extraordinary changes in my attitude toward life and death as a result of the experience. I appreciate my family much more. All my senses have been honed and sharpened. Above all, I have overcome many of my fears of dying because I'm enjoying life."

We can do several things to overcome our fears about death. First, we must realize that we cannot escape death. By accepting our coming death as a fact, we can neutralize the demoralizing and paralyzing fears. When we have a clear understanding of this fact, acceptance comes easier without false hopes or bitterness. Then we can really start living.

Second, after accepting the inevitability of death, we can become courageous, decisive, and fearless. We must assume a total plan for life, one which will help us to better understand that facing up to death leads to strength. To accept that death will come means to take charge of one's life.

Third, when we accept the fact that we will die, we waste no time finding meaning and fulfillment in life. When we live life fully, we fear death least and love life most. Once, when I was serving as a pallbearer, I came to see in a profound way, as we were carrying the casket to the open grave, that someday someone would be doing this for me. I realized then that I must make my time count between now and when I die.

As we establish continuity of life, we begin to understand that death only destroys the physical body. Physical death frees the spirit. Jesus Christ put it this way: "I have come that they [man] may have life, and have it to the full" (John 10:10). Paul wrote, "For to me, to live is Christ and to die is gain" (Philippians 1:21). A strong faith in God will equip us to overcome our fears of death and dying.

ELEVEN
STYLES OF DYING

From my teaching experience in a state university, I have become acquainted with several perspectives or styles of living and dying. The topics of dying, death, and the afterlife are faddish on most university campuses today. As one of my students said, "Death and the afterlife are extremely important to all of us because the birth rate and death rate are still one per person."

PHILOSOPHIES OF LIFE
Four major philosophical perspectives may be observed today concerning living and dying.

1. *Materialism.* The materialist rejects the idea that anything exists that cannot be weighed or measured. According to the philosophy of materialism, information and knowledge are restricted to only what can be perceived by our five physical senses. The materialist says that we cannot "know" nonmaterial objects, and since we cannot know nonmaterial things, we must reasonably conclude that they do not exist. To the materialist, it is a waste of time to try to discuss words such as *God*

and *soul* because meaning is reduced to knowing only material objects.

The materialist wants us to accept that everything came from nothing; order came from chaos; life came from nonlife; and morality came from amorality. To this, one young lady in my class once said, "It takes more faith to believe those claims than to believe in a personal, infinite, rational God who created the universe." I agree.

2. *Annihilationism.* According to this theory, wicked people pass into nonexistence and good people pass into soul-sleep when they die. Some of the cults today hold to this view.

As pressures of liberalism within Christianity continue, there will probably be more people moving toward the view of annihilationism. This philosophical view has come due to a weak view of Scripture being taught more and more today. This view has been expressed in many churches that do not teach that man has a soul that survives him at the death of the body. This view, in other words, reduces man to being only a body. Most biblical theologians conclude that annihilationism is based on false assumptions and reasoning. It seems regrettable that every few generations these arguments must come to be debated and answered all over again. Each time the proponents of annihilationism try to convince others that the Christian church has never dealt with these issues openly and fairly.

3. *Universalism.* Some believe that after death all people find themselves ultimately in an eternal state of bliss. Universalists have the sentimental idea that there is no such place as hell because God is too good to damn anyone. They view God as a kindly old grandfather with a "boys-will-be-boys" attitude, indifferent and powerless about evil and wrong in the world. In other words, they just *hope* that God will not judge people for their sins.

Believing that there is no punishment for sin, universalists teach that all people will go to heaven when they die, and that the suffering here on earth cleanses the wicked from their sins. Such a belief might seem pleasant and comforting, but it is not scripturally accurate. The Bible gives both good news and bad news. The message of the Scriptures is that "whoever believes . . . shall have eternal life," and "whoever does not believe stands condemned . . . because he has not believed in the name of God's one and only Son" (John 3:16, 18).

Universalism denies a final irreversible judgment. Someone said, "The brilliant jewels of eternal salvation can only be appreciated upon the black background of eternal punishment of those who reject God. In other words, the grace of God can be appreciated only to the extent that people understand the depth of God's wrath against sin.

4. *Historical Christianity.* This perspective presents the true Christian answer to life and death as found in the Scriptures. The Christian position views human nature in the complicated question, "What is man in relationship to past, present, and future?"

The Bible describes man as having a dual nature. Man cannot be reduced to being just a physical being or just a spiritual being but is, in some sense, both. The Bible teaches that man was created in the image of God. When man dies, his conscious mind survives the death of the physical body. According to his choices, man then either enjoys the bliss of God's presence or suffers eternal absence from God.

STYLES OF DYING

According to a person's philosophical or theological perspective, he develops a style of living and dying. A person's style of dying is inherent in his style of living. A person's attitudes about illness, dying, and death depend on his systems of beliefs. In recent years a book was written about how to live until death. The book, however, was more of an explanation of death. The author showed that there are at least six distinctly different ways of looking at death.[1]

Style One: "For everything there is a season." Such an accepting life-style meets death as an inevitable part of creation. It sees death as a natural part of life and says, "I accept it, actively or passively. But the important part is that I know it will happen. Any negative distress I try to set up only frustrates me. Therefore, the only sensible response is acceptance. As the Bible says, 'For everything there is a season.' "

Mortality cannot be denied. Death is common to all life on earth. For the person of traditional faith, death is not an end but a transition from one state of existence to another. It certainly is true that death is a part of the natural order of life and must be accepted.

The person who is accepting of death as a part of life would express his philosophy in the prayer used widely by Alcoholics Anonymous: "God, grant me the serenity to accept the things that I cannot change, the courage to change the things that I can, and the wisdom to know the difference."

Style Two: "Do not go gentle into that good night." Looking at death in this way would be someone who defies or rebels against death, seeing it as a personal destroyer. "There are many things inevitable in life, yet that does not mean that I have to wait and let them happen," such a person would say. "Death does not have a 'right' to take me. I will fight it every step of the way. When something important is taken from me, I feel cheated. It is not my task to make it easier on anyone. After all, I am the one who is 'paying' for death. I will show death a thing or two before it conquers me."

The person who holds this view realizes that dying is a natural and predictable part of life. Birth causes such a person to celebrate, but death is a dreaded and sorrowful time to be avoided by any means possible. Death reminds them of vulnerability.

There have been great technological advances, and death can be delayed, but not escaped. Even though people with this attitude fight death with all their might, they can never satisfy their desire to conquer it.

Style Three: "Eat, drink, and be merry." One with this sensuous life-style would fear death as the denial of human meaning. A happy, full life to him is good, but death negates the chance of continuing forever. "I will have a happy good time today and try never to worry about death," he would say. "I delight in pleasurable experiences even if great risks are involved. Sometimes the risks of good times make it even better for now."

The person who practices this philosophy usually thinks about dying only when he is forced to acknowledge death. He delights in experiences so he "parties" all the time in order to enjoy life now.

Hedonism is a word that adequately describes the life-style of such a person. The contemporary playboy philosophy is the clearest portrayal of this view of life. Everything in such a person's life is geared toward self-gratification and the denial of absolute values. Someone put this philosophy into words by saying, "I realize that someday I am going to die, but between now and then I am going to have the best time possible. When I am dead, I am dead. So I am going to enjoy as much sensual gratification as I can before I die."

Style Four: "No one ever dies with warm feet." This humorous expression is of a life-style that dances with death as around the edges of ultimate mystery. The philosophy behind this idea is if someone can laugh at death, he can conquer it. We discussed this attitude earlier in the book in describing how some people try to overcome their fear of death.

Death to such a person may be considered as the most serious subject in life. However, death, like any other subject, is not immune to humor. For the person with this attitude, having fun and being humorous whenever possible is a habit. Humor, when handled well, is constructive and enjoyable, but people who laugh at death see little else but humor in all aspects of it, from doctor-patient relationships to the funeral and even the afterlife. Some people challenge and make fun of death in an attempt to prove their superiority over it. Some of their jokes are innocent because they are an end in themselves and serve no particular aim. For example, someone told about the two young girls who were discussing their families. "Why does your grandmother read the Bible so much?" asked one. "I think she is cramming for her finals!" the other responded.

In a similar vein, someone said that when Thoreau was dying, he was asked, "Henry, have you made peace with God?" His reply was, "I did not know that we had ever quarreled."

The opposite kind are the aggressive jokes, the type people tell in order to try to assert their superiority over death. An example is the cynical one-liner: "The living are the dead on holiday."

In most cases, the people with this attitude about dying use jokes as a defense mechanism. A psychologist once described it: "Humor is a release of the unpleasant, transforming itself into pleasure." This satirical approach to life was expressed in the story of a Chicago gangster named Appel, who was condemned to be executed for murder. On the way to the electric chair, he turned to the newspaper reporters and said, "Stick around, gentleman, and you will soon see a baked Appel."

Style Five: "Good night, sweet prince." This tragic lifestyle sees death at any age coming always too soon. To someone with this attitude, everyone's death is premature. "Life is so very short even at its longest, I certainly cannot do all the things I want to do," they would say.

This philosophy, stated in the lines of Shakespeare's *Hamlet*, sees comedy always turning eventually into tragedy.

The people who embrace this view would agree with the famous Ernest Hemingway quote, "Every true story ends in death." For them, every experience is melancholic because they capitalize on the unfairness of life. One of my friends once demonstrated this style as she said, "I can enjoy life, but always against the backdrop of eventual death for myself and loved ones." Things may be going fine, but such people feel that sooner or later the fun and comedy of life will turn into tragedy and death. They never really enjoy living because they are obsessed with the fact that one day death will come.

Style Six: "Come now, greatest of feasts." Those of this life-style seek to find in death the meaning of existence. "I certainly will not give up my search for meaning in life as I am dying," they would say. "After all, I have even greater anticipation of finding meaning in death and after death."

Those of this view believe that all they have done and all that they are is culminated in their death. If they are fortunate enough to have advance notice that they are dying, then they get a final chance to grow. Death to them is a time to become all that they are meant to be.

These people usually encourage others not to wait until they find out they are dying to start to really live. They see death as an invisible, friendly companion on life's journey, who gently reminds them not to wait until later to do what they mean to do. It is through this philosophy of life and death that they realize that "living" is more than just simply passing time or existence.

These people not only rejoice at the opportunity of experiencing each new day, but are preparing for an ultimate acceptance of death. They desire to make their transition from life on earth to eternal life as the greatest "feast" of all times.

This group of people treats death as meaningful, as a growth-inducing aspect of life. They realize that dying is a process that people do continuously, not just at the end of physical life on earth. One of my friends put it this way: "If you can accept your death, perhaps you can learn to face and deal productively with each change during your life."

We have all probably known someone from each of these styles of living and dying. Perhaps the greatest question to ask ourselves is, "Have I directly or indirectly realized my own personal life-style of dying?" Regardless of one's perspective, it is probably not the dying that is so hard. Dying takes no skill or understanding. It can be done by anyone at any time. It is living that is hard. We must learn to live until we die. Whether our death is imminent or far away, we must love and live life fully.

TWELVE
SUICIDE

One afternoon in my office I listened to a college freshman cry his heart out. "I neither want to live or to die, but to do both at the same time—usually one more than the other," he said. One day he decided that he wanted to die more than he wanted to live.

Suicide is generally defined as the act of willfully causing one's own death in order to escape a condition of living that is perceived as intolerable. Another study defined suicide as the fatal act of self-injury, consciously or subconsciously undertaken with the intent of self-destruction. The cause and circumstances may be clear, vague, or ambiguous, yet the outcome is the death of self by one's own choosing.

Death from natural causes has its share of emotional overtones and torment, but suicide is seemingly the saddest and cruelest of all deaths. It presents the greatest of all affronts to those who survive. Much of life is directly or indirectly set in motion by factors beyond our control, but one of the most painful acts occurs when a close friend or relative takes his own life.

Suicide has always been a worldwide problem. In early Rome, suicide was considered honorable. Some of the Stoics and Epicureans suggested it as an alternative to the emptiness of life. The philosopher Socrates took poison rather than be exiled. In Europe prior to the twentieth century, suicide was a way to redeem oneself from class disgrace. Yet, in some civilizations, suicide was considered shameful. The countries that currently report the highest suicide rate are Finland, Denmark, Sweden, Hungary, West Germany, Austria, Japan, and the United States. Professionals tend to agree that in America for every one suicide there are eight to ten attempts.

A study of suicide reveals that people of every age, sex, religion, race, and social and economic class take their lives. It is the leading cause of unnecessary and stigmatizing death.

MYTHS ABOUT SUICIDE

Several widespread myths and false beliefs exist about people who are suicidal. The following are some of the most common.

1. Only crazy people or the insane would commit suicide.

2. If a person talks about killing himself, he will not commit suicide.

3. If a person makes a nonserious attempt to commit suicide, he will not try later to make a more serious attempt.

4. Someone living the good life—great home, good job, nice friends, money in the bank—will not attempt suicide.

5. Suicide is an inherited tendency.

6. If a person is under professional care, he will not commit suicide.

7. Only a specific class of people will commit suicide.

8. Suicide has simple causes that are basic in nature.

9. When a person who is suicidal starts to show improvement in behavior, the real danger is over.

It is possible that some of us and our friends and family believe a few of these myths. Perhaps some of us feel better when we learn that even some professionals also believe them to be true.

Self-destructive or suicidal people are categorized in one of the following three ways: (1) Those who threaten suicide by talking about it and have made some vague or unspecific plans; (2) those who attempt suicide, who consciously and deliberately put their plans into action, but for some reason do not successfully complete it; and (3) those who complete, consciously or unconsciously, the self-inflicted act.

The road to suicide begins with the first attempt or threat and ends in one's death. Family and friends are often confused about the cause or causes, and feelings of guilt and faultfinding are common among survivors. Of all the grief one can experience, there is perhaps none so difficult as the sorrow felt by family and friends when someone takes his own life. So many questions remain in the minds of the survivors! Everyone asks, "Why? What could I have done to prevent this? Did I show enough care and love?"

There are no easy or definite answers to any of these questions, since they could only have been answered by the one who died. The survivors are sincerely grieving for the one who consciously chose to end his or her life. For some reason, the person who committed suicide decided that he had encountered more pain than he could handle, so he decided to stop life on earth by means of death. It isn't that the person doesn't realize that his or her death will cause pain to others. Rather, he or she judges that his or her own pain is greater than everyone else's pain combined. It is the negative of discouragement, of seeing oneself as being of no use to anyone, that drives a person to suicide. Psychological evaluations following suicides show that most of the victims had directly or indirectly hinted for help from their physician, minister, social agent, or family. Yet, most of these caring people failed to recognize or understand the vague hints and intervene effectively.

Male suicide is usually due to a reaction to a loss of status, loss of a job or employment difficulties, or downward job mobility, resulting in a loss of desire to live. With women, suicide and suicide attempts are often a response to marital and romantic problems. Self-destructive behavior is an extreme response to a personal crisis. The pain and turmoil experienced by the person attempting suicide can be compared to the mixed feelings and confusion of someone trying to counsel and stop the act. In Judeo-Christian tradition, neither the Hebrew Old Testament or the New Testament dealt clearly or comprehensively with the rights or wrongs of suicide. There are several suicides recorded in the Bible:

Samson (Judges 16:30)
Saul and his armor bearer (1 Samuel 31:4, 5)
Ahithophel (2 Samuel 17:33)
Zimri (1 Kings 16:18)
Judas (Matthew 27:5)

An examination of these stories contributes little to a clear theology about suicide. Though it appears that God does not render a distinct judgment in any of these passages, it does not suggest in any way that suicide is desirable or commendable.

Over the years, suicide has taken on the character of being a deeply sinful act. Our feelings about suicide have deep historical roots. Among most people the suicide taboo is considered to be socially disgraceful and a moral offense.

Although the Bible does not make any precise statements about suicide, some people point to the letter of the law and say that the commandment "Thou shalt not kill" applies also to suicide—that is, if it is wrong to kill someone else, it is wrong to kill oneself. Others, who consider themselves apart from tradition, point out the spirit of the law of God's love and mercy toward those who have trusted him.

In the first part of the Bible, we read the thesis that has echoed throughout the centuries: "God saw all that he had made, and it was very good" (Genesis 1:31). Life is good. We should treasure it and never despair of its possibilities. In contemporary times, we are seeing that suicide is not only a spiritual question but also a major psychological and medical problem. Those who commit suicide may be sick in one or all of these areas: physical, resulting from some body chemistry imbalance; mental or intellectual status, suffering on an emotional or feelings level; and as the result of spiritual oppression. Suicidal people can be grouped in at least four psychological types.

1. The escapist—avoider. This type of person is trying to avoid some immediate difficulty or an intolerable situation. Another form of escapism is a suicide following the death of a significant person, producing what is considered an intolerable grief.

2. The aggressive—assertive. This type of person is seeking vengeance by inflicting remorse or pain on others. Another example of an aggressive suicide would be the person who commits a crime and then takes his life to cover up or keep from paying for his actions. Sometimes the aggressive suicide is done as a message to others of one's desperate predicament.

3. The sacrificial suicide. This type of person tries to gain some value greater than life. Such people commit suicide as a sacrifice in order to bring about some desired end, something that means more to them than life. Some suicides are by people trying to achieve some state

of delight, a kind of transfiguration experience.

4. The risker. This person is often involved in some great ordeal. He risks his life in order to prove something to himself in an issue. Another form of risking is related to game playing. A person may take a chance or gamble with death, as in so-called Russian roulette, placing a cartridge in only one chamber of a revolver, placing the revolver to the head, and pulling the trigger, gambling that the hammer will not fall on the loaded chamber.

MOTIVES

Regardless of the type of suicide, motives may fit into such categories as:

1. A signal of distress, given with the hope that some-one will intervene with help.

2. A signal of reactions to feelings of inner disintegration.

3. A signal to manipulate someone by punishing them.

4. A signal of anger toward another person. Such anger is internalized as guilt and depression.

5. A signal of a desire to join a deceased person who was significant to the person threatening suicide.

Those who take their own lives often leave notes. Sociologists have suggested that there are basically four kinds. One kind of note gives directions to the survivors. This type almost becomes a last will and testament, in that it gives instructions. The letter is usually personal, telling what should be done with possessions.

A second kind of note presents oneself as an innocent bystander. In this note the person usually asks for forgiveness and tries to show that the ones to whom the note was written were not responsible for what happened. Then the note gives a reason why it was necessary to take his or her life and acknowledges that the survivors will probably not understand.

A third type of suicide note is written by a person who has or imagines that he has a terminal illness that will be extremely painful. This person assumes that the survivors will understand and readily forgive the action.

The fourth type of letter is written to blame something or someone for being responsible for the problems and circumstances that led to the suicide. It is usually brief and does not seek forgiveness or state reasons, but seeks only to blame others.

Often friends or relatives will discover a potential suicide's note before the act occurs. If such notes are found, one should always assume that the person who wrote it is serious and take some immediate and responsible action. Whatever one decides to do, it should be done quickly while there is time to save a life.

INDICATORS TO WATCH FOR
The following is a list revealing the most common indicators of potential suicide.

> Extremely low self-esteem
> Intense and continual expressions of unhappiness
> Hopelessness concerning a situation
> Previous suicide attempts
> Statements of suicide intent
> Giving away most valuable possessions
> Placing final affairs in order
> Breakdown or absence of support system
> Extreme rebellious behavior
> Breakdown of health
> Neglect of responsibilities
> Severe or sudden personality changes

The ability to comprehend and cope with depression and difficulties in life appears to be a learned behavior. Most suicidal people are not willing to wait for life to teach them that their feelings are normal and can be handled.

Suicide is such a complex behavior that it is exceptionally difficult to prevent or control. Those who study suicide say that invariably the act is associated with some sense of loss. The losses may be emotional. The loss of a significant relationship such as a spouse or child may cause a person to become suicidal. The loss may be psychological. The loss of self-esteem or confidence may cause a person to want to die. It may be a physical problem, as the loss of a limb or of good health, which may discourage a person from wanting to live, since he feels he won't ever be normal again. The loss may be social, as the loss of a best friend or of a cherished neighborhood. Social pressures may become unbearable and cause a person to decide that life is not worth living.

Suicidal people tend to magnify the question of quality or quantity of life. When a person decides that quality has depreciated too much, he no longer wants to live, especially when a crisis arises. Those who still see a glimmer of hope will usually seek help. Those who don't are likely to want to kill themselves quickly.

The real tragedy is that many of these people could probably cope successfully with any one of their problems if the problems were isolated long enough to be resolved one by one. But when problems seem too big or too many to handle at one time, the result may be suicide. Several other things must be kept in mind concerning those who commit suicide. For example, the one who committed suicide probably did not do it to others—he did it to solve some of his own problems. His suicide means that life became too painful and unbearable for him. Consciously or unconsciously, he determined to stop life on earth. The alternative of death seemed to him better than living.

We must not "judge . . . lest [we] be judged" (Matthew

7:1). When a suicide occurs, most families and friends are judgmental and condemning. We must be careful not to present simple answers to complex problems. We must relate to others with compassion and understanding, since we do not fully comprehend all the problems and pressures that the person who died endured in life. Everyone has a breaking point. Some people have more difficulty in responding to circumstances and stress pressures. It is not fair for survivors to blot out the memory of a life because of one final tragic act.

We should also remember that there is hope in salvation. The question always comes up, "Can a person go to heaven if he commits suicide?" Salvation, according to the Scriptures, is not based on the way we die, but on a person's faith, which results in a relationship with God through Jesus Christ. The Apostle Paul wrote, "For it is by grace you have been saved, through faith—and this not from yourselves, it is the gift of God—not by works, so that no one can boast" (Ephesians 2:8, 9). The manner of a person's death does not enter into the picture. Nothing—not even death—can separate us from the love of God which is in Christ Jesus.

Certain ideas about suicide can be summarized from contemporary theological, sociological, and psychological writings. First, suicide is always criticized; but there is a desire to understand and to pity victims of suicide. Second, no one seems to want to condemn but to fight against suicide by attacking the major causes. The causes are usually neuroses, loneliness, and depression. The problem is recognized as being far more theological and psychological than sociological.

When a suicide occurs, the survivors' grief is a major crisis. As they go through the normal grief process, they have a tendency to find someone to blame for the suicide. This desire arises from the feelings of helplessness and guilt in not having been able to prevent the suicide.

Sometimes a survivor will go to the extreme and deny that the suicide took place, perhaps the only way he or she can handle the situation. Usually the grieving survivor pretends or insists that the death was an accident. The family and close friends of a suicide victim pay an especially high price from the aftereffects if they do not get support during this time of crisis.

Survivors of suicide victims need to make an effort to forgive the deceased and also the living for what happened. As best they can, they must realize that the victim responded out of deep mental, emotional, physical, and perhaps spiritual pain. Others must forgive the survivors for not realizing the intensity of pain or immediacy of the dead person's situation. A suicide presents a great challenge to survivors to forgive the victim for denying them a chance to respond to his needs. All those involved must forgive themselves and each other for each other's inadequacies.

Perhaps someone is thinking and feeling, "But I cannot forgive them." Forgiveness is a commitment that is made to ourselves and others. Not by what we think or feel, but by an act of our will we choose to make the commitment to forgive. After this commitment is made, thoughts and feelings will follow—sometimes much later. If we are unable to forgive, we will never experience real life with any quality.

It is too late to do anything about a suicide after the fact, but there is much we can do to prevent future suicides. Professionals who work with suicidal people agree that such people are calling for help and trying to tell us something by their behavior. We usually get what we need by asking for it. But suicidal people usually do not know how to ask openly for help. Such cries for help are generally stated in one of the following ways:

"Please save me from myself."

"Please help me to find something to live for."

"Please stop me from killing myself."

Yet, these messages are rarely stated that clearly. Usually the statements are much more indirect, such as:

"There is nothing in life left for me since my husband left me."

"This pain is too much. I can't take it anymore. I must stop it."

"I cannot live without my girlfriend. Nobody will ever be able to take her place."

"I cannot take these problems anymore."

"I do not want to die, nor do I want to live. I don't know which I want most."

Many suicides could have been prevented if only the problem had been recognized. One complicating factor is that, on the surface, suicidal people seem little different from other people. Another hindrance to solutions is that some people seem fearful of approaching suicide education, thinking that the study of it might cause some people to think more about the subject, which would in turn produce a rash of suicides. Fortunately, others today are realizing that in order to deal with any problem there must be an openness toward truth.

GUIDELINES

There is no magic formula to dealing with potential suicides. Yet, a few guidelines should be followed:

1. Take the suicide statement seriously. At the same time, do not panic or give an exaggerated response to the one who is considering suicide.

2. Do not provoke the person who is thinking about suicide. Many times, by saying the wrong things, we can intensify the suicidal desire.

3. Listen—really listen—to what the potential suicidal person is trying verbally and nonverbally to say. Suicidal people can discern whether someone really cares and is

on their side or whether he is just humoring them, stalling for time, or trying some other form of manipulation.

4. Know appropriate resource persons available in your location. Do not try to be a "lone ranger" in helping a potential suicide. Seek the assistance of others who are capable of joining you in your effort to save life.

5. Create an aura of hope. One fact is characteristic of every suicide—the person has lost hope and looks at life as a hopeless mess. Do not confirm his pessimism. All our hope is not restricted to life after death. Jesus Christ offers practical hope and help for facing problems in this present life.

Beyond these suggestions, there are several practical things that we should do when we perceive that someone is suicidal. As mentioned earlier, do not ignore his behavior. Focus on his particular crisis by listening and asking questions. Sometimes we also have to listen to what is not being said. When you realize that a person is perhaps contemplating suicide, ask some questions, such as:

"Are you thinking about suicide?" If he is, he will probably tell you. If he is not, he will say, "Oh, no!"

"How long have you been thinking like this?" The answer will give further clues as to how serious he is. Watch also for nonverbal behavior for part of the answer.

"How would you do it? What is your plan?" If the person can tell you a definite plan, you know he is very serious.

"How angry are you?" The answer may give you some clues to problem areas. It will give a suicidal person an opportunity to vent his anger and hurt.

"Why do you want to die?" As you listen to the response, you may be able to determine whether you need to make a referral. As you talk with a suicidal person using these questions, continue to interpret the nonverbal communication—what he is not saying. If you are not comfortable with your competence in helping, make a referral to a professional you can trust.

A letter was once written to a famous advice columnist, Ann Landers. Her response gives the general attitude of the public toward suicide:

> Dear Ann: Why can't a person leave this world when he is ready by simply taking a pill and going to sleep forever? I am sure many people would welcome such a blessed release. Why haven't doctors thought of this? When animals suffer, it is considered merciful to put them to sleep. I believe every doctor should be permitted to give his patients the same consideration animals get. Don't you? (signed) A Reader in St. Louis.

> Dear Reader: Thousands of people do exactly what you have suggested every year. It's called suicide. The flaw in your reasoning is this: Many pills can be obtained by prescription only because people must be protected against killing themselves while in a depressed state or at a time when they are suffering temporary physical or emotional distress.

> Many people who are enjoying life today will tell you there have been times when they would have taken a handful of pills if they had had them—and it's a good thing they didn't. Death is permanent.[1]

At some time in our lives we may need some general knowledge about suicide crisis intervention. If the town where you live does not have a suicide phone hotline, you should call the local hospital emergency room for assistance and referral. Community mental health centers usually have hotlines or walk-in care centers.

Across the nation are large centers that may be called from anywhere, day or night. These centers are prepared to help or refer anyone to a help center in the appropriate geographic location.

Below is a list of major centers in America:

Suicide Prevention Center
1041 South Menlo
Los Angeles, CA 90006
213-386-5111

Suicide Prevention Center of San Mateo County
1811 Trousdale Drive
Burlingame, CA 94010
San Mateo North 415-877-5600
Belmont South 415-367-8000
Coastside 415-726-5228

Alachua County Crisis Center
606 S.W. Third Avenue
Gainesville, FL 32601
904-376-4444

Baton Rouge Crisis Intervention Center, Inc.
P. O. Box 80738
Baton Rouge, LA 70898
504-924-3900

Life Crisis Services, Inc.
7438 Forsyth, Suite 210
St. Louis, MO 63105
314-725-2010

National Save-a-Life League
4520 Fourth Avenue, Suite MH3
Brooklyn, NY 11220
718-491-4067

Suicide Prevention Center, Inc.
184 Salem Avenue
Dayton, OH 45406
513-223-4777

Crisis Intervention Center
P. O. Box 120934
Nashville, TN 37212
615-244-7444

Suicide and Crisis Center
2910 Swiss Avenue
Dallas, TX 75209
214-828-1000

Crisis Intervention of Houston
P. O. Box 13066
Houston, TX 77219
713-228-1505

Crisis Clinic
1530 Eastlake East
Seattle, WA 98102
206-447-3222

The Samaritans
Boston, MA
617-247-0220

Falmouth, MA
617-548-8900

Lawrence, MA
617-688-6607

Keene, NH
603-357-5505

Providence, RI
401-272-4044

Chicago, IL
312-947-8300

New York City
212-664-0505

If you desire more information about beginning a peer
counseling group, you may write or call:

Youth Rescue Fund
3575 Cahuenga Boulevard West
Suite 255
Los Angeles, CA 90068
213-850-3323

Youth Rescue Fund
6715 Lowell Avenue
McLean, VA 22101
703-237-7950

PART III
GRIEF

THIRTEEN
THE FUNERAL
OR MEMORIAL SERVICE

Society marks life's significant events with appropriate ceremonies. For example, we celebrate birthdays with parties, we hold graduation exercises, marriage ceremonies, and we celebrate anniversaries. Death, one of life's most significant events, is marked by funeral or memorial services.

The funeral industry defines a funeral as an organized and purposeful, time-limited, flexible, group-centered response to death. The funeral is a ceremony during which relatives, friends, and associates give their respects to the deceased and their comfort to the survivors. Funerals usually span a period of two to four days. In most instances the event takes place in the presence of the deceased body.

The funeral observance usually begins with a time of visitation of the survivors, held at the funeral home or at the home of the deceased. The visitation is followed by the funeral or memorial service, conducted either in a church, funeral chapel, or public auditorium. Following the service, there is the committal or interment at the cemetery or mausoleum. The observance is often concluded with a gathering at the house of worship, at the home of the deceased, some public meeting place, or at the home of a member of the surviving family.

There is no one prescribed form for a funeral or memorial service. The survivors, the minister, and the funeral director can arrange whatever kind of service that best meets the family's needs and desires.

During the funeral period there are many ways in which people may share in the survivors' loss and express their love, respect, and grief. Some people will come to both the visitation and the funeral or memorial service. Others may attend just one. Most of those who attend the funeral service will also be present at the committal or interment. Some of those who come to be with the bereaved during this time as well as those who could not attend also express their sympathy by offering comfort and consolation by sending flowers, plants, or some other form of remembrance. Some families consider gifts of flowers a waste and will, with the funeral announcement, designate a charitable organization to which gifts in memory of the deceased may be sent in lieu of flowers.

The funeral or memorial service is held in memory of the person who has died but is for the survivors. This is why it is important for the relatives, friends, and associates to accept expressions of empathy. Such expressions are beneficial to the receiver as well as the giver.

WHAT A FUNERAL SERVICE SHOULD BE

1. The funeral service must deal with death realistically.

2. The funeral service must present a vision of God which will be of comfort and help to mourners in their suffering. This includes the understanding of the love of

God, the nearness of God, and God's concern for his people.

3. The service must see man as an individual of value, worth, and dignity. Attention should be turned to the importance of the resources God offers to strengthen and stabilize us at such a difficult time.

4. The service must demonstrate that the Christian faith is a resource that allows and enables the individual to mourn, rather than a cause of denial or a substitute for mourning.

5. The service must recognize and accept deep feelings rather than cover them up by a superficial aestheticism.

6. The service must provide a sense of finality.

7. The service must be an aid in recalling memories of the deceased.

8. The service must establish a proper climate for mourning.

9. The service must be planned in such a way as to be sensitive to the individual needs of the bereaved.

WHAT A FUNERAL SERVICE SHOULD DO

1. The funeral or memorial service should provide a reinforcement for the reality of death and dying.

2. It should provide a framework of supportive community of relationships for the survivors.

3. It should provide a ritual that is intended to convey the Christian meaning of life and death, presenting a consistent view of both in the context of faith.

4. It should provide an outlet for the mourners to give expression of authentic emotions.

5. It should provide an affirmation of the meaning of the life that has been lived.

6. It should provide a ceremony that marks a fitting conclusion to the life of the deceased.

KINDS OF SERVICES

There are several alternatives to the traditional funeral. Many people do not realize the following alternatives are available:

1. A memorial service involving rites, ceremonies, and commemoration without the body being present. In this case, the disposition of the body has already taken place prior to the service or will take place later with no one in attendance except the functionaries involved.

2. A grave-side service only. Such a service has all the rites or ceremonies at the grave-side prior to the committal. There is no viewing of the body, no visitation, and no service at a church or funeral chapel.

3. A direct disposition without rites or ceremonies. The body is taken from the place of death to the funeral home or other facilities where it must be kept as long as required by law and to allow time for necessary papers to be processed. Then the body is taken to the place of disposition.

4. There are some who desire to donate their body to medical science and have no funeral. Others choose to have the usual visitation and a memorial service after the body has been donated to science.

Regardless of the kind of service, it should be a victorious expression, one that gives opportunity to focus on the reality of death in the midst of a supportive community.

REGULATION OF THE FUNERAL INDUSTRY

The funeral profession is regulated in the United States by two sources: state and federal laws, and regulations self-imposed by the funeral trade associations themselves. The following codes of professional standards must be met by morticians and funeral homes.

Code of Ethics,[1] National Funeral Directors' Association of the United States, Inc.

I

As funeral directors, we herewith fully acknowledge our individual and collective obligations to the public, especially to those we serve, and our mutual responsibilities for the proper welfare of the funeral service profession.

II

To the public we pledge: vigilant support of health laws; proper legal regulations for the members of our profession; devotion to high moral and service standards; conduct befitting good citizens; honesty in all offerings of service and merchandise, and in all business transactions.

III

To those we serve we pledge: confidential business and professional relationships; cooperation with the customs of all religions and creeds; observance of all respect due the deceased; high standards of competence and dignity in the conduct of all services; truthful representation of all services and merchandise.

IV

To our profession we pledge: support of high educational standards and proper licensing laws; encouragement of scientific research; adherence to sound business practices; adoption of improved techniques; observance of all rules of fair competition; maintenance of favorable personnel relations.

When death occurs, the person responsible for the funeral should be advised to contact his family funeral director or direct that he be notified as soon as possible. This should be done regardless of where or when death takes place. The funeral director then becomes the representative of the family for the purpose of the funeral arrangements.

When the funeral director is called by the family or their representative, he arranges to remove the body and to provide the necessary services and materials in keeping with the wishes and finances of the family or their representative.

Before any funeral arrangements are made, the funeral director should determine, if he does not know, who is the minister, priest, or rabbi of the deceased and family. The funeral director should make certain that the clergyman has been notified about the death. If it hasn't been done, the funeral director should suggest it be done or offer to do so himself.

The specifics and all aspects of the religious part of the funeral should be discussed and cleared with the clergyman. These arrangements may be done either by the family or the funeral director or both.

Before the family selects the funeral services, the funeral director should explain the various aspects of the funeral, the costs of the services and wares he provides, the cost of the services, such as cemeteries, and florists. This discussion of prices should take place before the family goes into the casket selection room. The funeral director, in his presentation, should make clear the range of prices of funerals he has available. He should also welcome any questions or discussions about what is or is not required by law.

The funeral director should review for the family the various death benefits or burial allowances that may be available to them through Social Security, the Veterans Administration, labor unions, or other fraternal organizations. He should assist in the preparation and filing of the necessary forms to secure these benefits and allowances for the family. Where further professional assistance is required, he should be prepared to make some recommendations as to where the family can secure such help.

Because the total price of the funeral is related to the casket selection, there should be a card or brochure in each casket in the selection room. Such a card or brochure should outline the services offered by the funeral home. Services and merchandise not included, where a unit price method is used, should be listed on the card or brochure as separate items.

The funeral director, in discussing caskets, should describe the material, construction, design, hardware, mattressing, and interior. He should explain the construction, design, and use of outside receptacles in which the casketed body is placed and any requirements of cemeteries as to the use of such receptacles.

When a family decides on the kind of service desired, the funeral director should provide a memorandum or agreement for the family to approve or sign showing (1) the price of the service that the family has selected and what it includes; (2) the price of each of the supplemental items of service and materials requested; (3) the amount involved for each of the items for which the funeral director will advance monies as an accommodation to the family; and (4) the method of payment agreed upon by the family and the funeral director.

When death occurs in a place other than where the funeral or burial are to take place, usually the services of two funeral directors are necessary. Under such circumstances the family should not pay for a complete service at both places.

The forwarding funeral director and the receiving director should coordinate their services and charges and make a written report to the family. This practice insures that neither funeral director charges the family for the services already provided by the other.

As soon as the details and schedule in the transporting of the remains are known to the forwarding funeral director, he is responsible for notifying and coordinating details with the receiving director. When a body is going to be transported, the person who did the embalming should prepare a written report that will accompany the body, explaining whatever professional services have already been done. Such a report will be of assistance to the receiving funeral director in the event additional work needs to be done.

If the burial is held in some city other than where the funeral service is conducted, the concrete or metal burial vault to be used should be arranged for by the director responsible for the interment to eliminate the added handling and transportation costs.

When a funeral service is conducted in a place other than the church of the clergyman, his wishes and desires should be considered to whatever extent possible.

In the matter of the honorarium or stipend, the wishes of the clergyman should be respected. If the family is a member of the clergyman's church or parish, it is a personal matter between the family and the clergyman. When the funeral director assumes the responsibility for the honorarium at the direction of the family, it is desirable to use a check for the transaction for record-keeping purposes. If the clergyman does not accept honoraria, the family should be so informed in order that they may express their appreciation in other ways. When the family makes no choice of a clergyman, and if the funeral director makes arrangement for one, the matter of who pays the honorarium becomes the responsibility of the funeral director.

When conducting a funeral in a church, the policy of that church must serve as the guide to the conduct of the service. Any exceptions to such procedures requested by the family should be cleared with the clergyman or church authorities well in advance of the time of their actual performance. The funeral director should remain alert to the needs of the families he serves and when the need for religious or pastoral counseling is indicated, he should make proper referrals.

Funeral directors should be available to discuss with anyone all matters relative to the conduct of a funeral. Whenever possible they should assume active leadership in seminars or discussions to bring about a deeper understanding about death, the funeral, and bereavement.

One of the groups in the funeral industry that I have found very cooperative is the National Selected Morticians. Their code of professional ethics given below is outstanding.

The Code of Good Funeral Practice, National Selected Morticians[2]

As funeral directors, our calling imposes upon us special responsibilities to those we serve and to the public at large. Chief among them is the obligation to inform the public so that everyone can make knowledgeable decisions about funerals and funeral directors.

In acceptance of our responsibilities, and as a condition of our membership in National Selected Morticians, we affirm the following standards of good funeral practice and hereby pledge:

1. To provide the public with information about funerals, including prices, and about the functions, services, and responsibilities of funeral directors.

2. To afford a continuing opportunity to all persons to discuss or arrange funerals in advance.

3. To make funerals available in as wide a range of price categories as necessary to meet the need of all segments of the community, and affirmatively to extend to everyone the right of inspecting and freely considering all of them.

4. To quote conspicuously in writing the charges for every funeral offered; to identify clearly the services, facilities, equipment, and merchandise included in such

quotations; and to follow a policy of reasonable adjustment when less than the quoted offer is utilized.

5. To furnish each family, at the time funeral arrangements are made, a written memorandum of charges and to make no additional charge without the approval of the purchaser.

6. To make no representation, written or oral, which may be false or misleading, and to apply a standard of total honesty in all dealings.

7. To respect all faiths, creeds, and customs, and to give full effect to the role of the clergy.

8. To maintain a qualified and competent staff, complete facilities, and suitable equipment required for comprehensive funeral service.

9. To assure those we serve the right of personal choice and decision in making funeral arrangements.

10. To be responsive to the needs of the poor, serving them within their means.

We pledge to conduct ourselves in every way and at all times in such a manner as to deserve the public trust, and to place a copy of this Code of Good Funeral Practice in the possession of a representative of all parties with whom we arrange funerals.

RESOURCES

The serious student of death education can obtain information about the funeral profession from the following associations:

American Certified Morticians Association
35 North Arroyo Parkway
Pasadena, CA 91109

Center for Death Education and Research
University of Minnesota
1167 Social Science Building
Minneapolis, MN 55455

Continental Association for Funeral
and Memorial Societies, Inc.
1828 L Street, N.W.
Suite 1100
Washington, DC 20036

Guild of American Funeral Directors
30112 Silver Spur Road
San Juan Capistrano, CA 92675

Jewish Funeral Directors of America, Inc.
3501 14th Street, N.W.
Washington, DC 20010

National Association of Coroners
and Medical Examiners
2121 Adelbert Road
Cleveland, OH 44106

The National Funeral Directors Association of the
United States, Inc.
135 North Wells Street
Milwaukee, WI 52103

National Selected Morticians
1616 Central Street
Evanston, IL 60201

A list of accredited schools of mortuary science can be
obtained from:

The American Board of Funeral Service Education, Inc.
201 Columbia Street
Fairmont, WV 26554

FOURTEEN
THE GRIEF
PROCESS
FOR SURVIVORS

Though human grief is too complex for simplistic labels, we will attempt to describe certain steps or stages of normal grief. One major reason people have trouble adjusting is that they do not understand the normal grief process. Because they don't understand it, they treat their grief as if it were something abnormal and feel that they themselves are abnormal or subnormal when grief overwhelms them.

People who have never had to confront the issue may not understand the adjustments to it. Despite the inevitability of death, bereavement usually seems to come unexpectedly. Since this is true, few people put forth any effort before the situation faces them to understand the normal process of grief.

It does not make any difference how brave and strong we are, or think we are. We must call grief or sorrow by its right name in order to comprehend it for what it is. A grieving person should not, by any reflection or twist of words, minimize what he is going through when death removes one of his family or friends. The fact remains— when someone who was loved by us is deceased, he is no longer with us and it is normal human reaction to

169

miss him. Grief is the process of readjustment to the environment from which the deceased person is now missing but in which we start forming new relationships.[1] In other words, it is a series of thoughts, feelings, and actions during a period of adjustment to the loss of a loved one. Most people are inadequate within themselves to cope with all the crisis situations surrounding death. In some ways, death might be more difficult for the bereaved than for the deceased.

When death occurs, there are several stages of grief for the mourning survivors. A survivor does not necessarily go through all the stages, nor does he necessarily go through them in the order in which they are presented here. Sometimes it is difficult to differentiate between the stages. The normal grief pattern may include shock, emotional strain, weeping, panic, depression, physical distress, guilt, resentment, repression, and hope.

1. *Shock*. Shock is a blow, impact, a sudden agitation of the mental or emotional sensibilities. It is a numbing, anesthetized reaction we may experience immediately upon hearing about the death of someone we love.

Shock may last a few minutes, hours, or days. If it goes on for weeks, then it becomes unhealthy. We should not be afraid of this initial period of shock. On several occasions when I have learned of the death of someone dear to me, I was stunned. I walked around in almost a trance or daze. I heard people talking to me, but the words did not register. I was numb.

Shock is a temporary escape from reality. It is also the body's natural way of protection and God's provision or gift to help us endure the initial effects of grief. After a few hours or days we must face the reality of the loss. One of the best things to do for someone in shock is to keep him busy carrying on as much normal activity as possible during the crisis time. The sooner the person has to deal with immediate problems and make decisions, the better. This may seem hard, but otherwise

they could lose a great deal of self-confidence and contact with reality. We should be near and available to
help, but should not hinder the therapeutic value to be
gained by the person's doing what he can do for himself.

A person's sense of shock may come and go. When in
shock I sometimes find myself saying, "I can't believe
this really happened." I know that it did happen, but at
first I can't accept it emotionally.

In addition to a mental shock, a sudden death brings
also a social shock. A married person is suddenly single.
To have to function socially all of a sudden without a
spouse is to experience some sense of shock.

2. *Emotions and weeping.* Emotions cannot be sepa-
rated from the situations or experiences that evoke
them. Emotion is an inside thermometer that registers
outside events. When a person is in grief, weeping is an
impulse expression of inner feelings. The first step in
dealing with weeping is to realize that it is an emotional
expression and that it is God's way of helping us to
relieve inner pressure.

When it begins to dawn upon us that we have lost
someone we love, these emotional feelings well up and
we feel the uncontrollable urge to express our grief. The
most healthy thing to do is to allow ourselves to weep
and truly express the emotions we feel.

In American society, it is difficult for some men to cry.
They have been taught very early, as little boys, "Men
do not cry." Therefore, many men think that weeping is
a sign of weakness or femininity. But people who tense
up and refuse to express their emotions may be in for
trouble. The expression of emotions is essential to most
people. For someone to try to repress his emotions is to
make himself less human.

Tears might be defined as "love drops," as we do not
weep for anything that is insignificant. To weep for
someone means that we care and love deeply.

In talking about emotions, we are not talking about

emotionalism. One of the faults of many so-called "spiritual robots" is that their perspective seems to have stifled the expressions of sorrow at the death of a loved one. We should encourage the expression of grief. Sometimes people are embarrassed to sorrow or weep openly. If this is the case, they should be allowed some solitude to let their sorrow take its natural course.

There are a number of ways in which we may release our emotions. We should not keep them bottled up within ourselves. We may express them to ourselves, to a friend, or to someone whom we know cares for us. There is truth in the idea that a joy shared doubles it; a sorrow shared halves it. An expression of grief may not be a once-for-all happening. It is normal to continue to weep at times about one's loss for a year or two. Significant days concerning the deceased are hard to face, such as birthdays, Mother's Day, or the anniversary of the death.

3. *Panic.* Panic is a sudden, severe, overpowering fright. When we are confronted or obsessed with a loss, in some instances we become panicky because we can think of nothing but the loss. When I am in the grief process my mind seems to go only a few seconds without thinking about my loss. The inability to concentrate is normal and natural at such times.

Fear of the unknown or fear of something that we do not understand causes us to panic. It is important that people understand the grief process before they experience it so that they will not treat such normal behavior as if it were abnormal. Knowledge of what happens normally during grief can eliminate part of the panic.

The first time I went through deep sorrow, I did not know what to expect. I thought that my life was a wreck because of the feelings that flooded me. I began to panic. I thought that I might even be losing my mind because I could not control my feelings, thoughts, or words.

Gloom soon surrounds panic. At such times it is natural to want to be alone. However, we must not linger in our gloom because it will only extend the adjustment time. It is a comfort to understand that even panic is a normal reaction to a stressful situation such as death.

4. *Depression.* Panic may soon turn into depression. In the normal grief process many people may eventually feel depressed. Depression is the saddening and lowering of mental spirit. It is the feeling resulting from an extreme difficulty or burden, an emotional state of dejection or despair, apprehension, and feelings of worthlessness.

When we find ourselves in depression or despair, we often feel that no one has ever had a loss as significant as ours. Then something seems to come between us, family, friends, and even God. We often find ourselves thinking thoughts that we would never otherwise have ventured. At one point in my deep sorrow, I felt that no one cared—not even God. I knew that God could have kept the death from happening if he would have wanted, but he did not. And I was angry. It is easy to get a "persecution complex" when we are depressed. One of the best things we can do for someone depressed in grief is to stand by him in quiet confidence and assure him that "this too shall pass." The bereaved person will probably not understand you at first, but later, as the depression lifts, he will.

For some people the depression clouds roll away in a day or two. For others it may take weeks and months before some ray of light breaks through.

5. *Physical distress.* If depression is prolonged, signs of physical and mental distress may appear. Physical distress is the result of physical pain and symptoms of illness arising from the grief process. Many people actually become physically ill because they have not worked through their grief. Emotional problems not resolved become physical problems. Notice I said "resolved," not "solved." One cannot solve the problem of the separa-

tion of a loved one by death. But to resolve the problem is to learn to live with the separation, to come to a reasonable acceptance and adjustment to the loss.

Some of the physical symptoms of distress during the grief process might be (a) feelings of tightness in the throat, (b) choking, with shortness of breath, (c) need for sighing, (d) empty feeling in the abdomen, (e) lack of muscular power, and (f) tension distress. A person in grief may be affected with horrible dreams that may emotionally drain him. Such physical and mental distress is normal unless it continues for too long.

6. *Guilt.* When a person feels distress and sorrow, he may also start feeling guilty. Guilt is normally the feeling of having committed a breach of conduct. Guilt comes when one does not meet what he expects of himself or what others expect of him. Neurotic guilt is guilt feelings out of proportion to the conduct.

Guilt feelings often come when someone feels that he should have been there to do or to suggest something that may have been of some comfort or assistance to the deceased.

Negative guilt feelings may come when one realizes that he did not treat the deceased properly. God's promise in 1 John 1:9 is a good prescription for guilt. "If we confess our sins [God] is faithful . . . and will forgive us our sins." Negative guilt feelings and misunderstood emotions make us miserable for a long time. We must not be afraid to talk about our feelings of guilt with those who care for us.

Often there is a feeling that one's responsibility to the loved one was not properly taken care of while the person was alive. Sometimes there is a basis for this, but on many occasions, this may not be true. Whatever the reason for the feelings of guilt, it should be realized that it is normal to feel guilty about situations which we desired to make better but couldn't.

7. *Repression.* When we can't make the situation bet-

ter, then feelings of resentment or repression may begin. Repression is a defense behavior by which someone prevents painful thoughts and desires from entering the conscious mind. It is, in other words, "selective forgetting." The thoughts are not really forgotten, for they keep coming back, in one form or another, to the conscious mind.

Repressed feelings continue to influence behavior. Often the person is unaware of the real basis for some of his thoughts, beliefs, and actions. A new painful experience may trigger a flood of many repressed feelings. If a person is trying to repress his feelings about the death of a loved one, and he suddenly sees a funeral procession, or perhaps even smells flowers that he has associated with the funeral of a loved one, or hears a favorite song of the loved one, he may break into tears. He could not continue to repress the painful feelings that were bottled up inside.

Repressed feelings or thoughts may be very active and may find an outlet in dreams when the conscious mind lowers its controls. When a person is under continued frustration, repressed thoughts may increase in strength and threaten to break through into the conscious mind and even into overt actions.

Threats of mentally painful experiences lead to the arousal of anxiety and additional defenses. Repression is a form of self-deception. It is much better to be realistic and work through the painful thoughts than to expend all the mental energy it takes to repress thoughts, energy that would be better directed toward attempts to resolve the problems of life.

Repressed feelings that are allowed to come into the conscious mind bring with them feelings of resentment.

8. *Resentment.* Resentment is the feeling of indignant displeasure because of something regarded as wrong. In our depression, strong feelings of hostility and resentment may arise.

Many who are in the grief process go through a time of being very critical of everything and everyone who was related to the loss. As one tries to understand why the death happened, he tends to blame others. He expresses resentment to anyone who cared for the patient. No matter what was done on behalf of the deceased, he feels that it was insufficient.

This type of resentment gives rise to questions like "Why did God let this happen?" We discussed earlier some of the answers to this question based on what we know of the laws of nature, human imperfection, community living, and divine impartiality. At times a person becomes so desperate in his resentment that he cannot live with himself, much less with anyone else. A resentful person hurts himself more than anyone else.

It is comforting to know that all such behavior within reasonable limits is normal in the grief process. In spite of resentment and all other emotions, there is hope.

9. *Hope/Acceptance.* Hope is the expectation of a comfortable new normal life. We need to express our emotions. We need encouragement from others. Some people think that in their grief, as a means of showing respect for the dead, they should shut out all possibilities for a new and meaningful normal life. Notice that I did not say "the old and meaningful normal life." The past is gone. Life will never be the same as we knew it with our loved ones. But there can be a "new normal life."

When I experienced the deep sorrow of the grief process for the first time, I felt I would never be happy again and that nothing could ever ease the heartache. I did not know that it was normal to feel that way for a while. Only in acceptance lies hope. There is no hope or peace in forgetting, nor in resignation, nor in busyness. Acceptance is the key. One may ask, "But how do I accept something that I don't want to accept?" We must be willing to let go of our selfish motives and trust God and his sovereignty. If we aren't, then we must keep praying for such a willingness to accept.

God is never weary with our new beginnings. We need to ask God for thoughts of mind and impressions of heart as we accept his ultimate sovereign plan for our lives. The Bible is a record of men who have taken God at his word and trusted. God does not always grant us our wants, desires, and wishes, but he does meet our needs. Many times I get the distinctions of words such as desires, wishes, wants, and needs mixed up. God meets our real needs as we trust him. Jesus comes to us at the point of our need and shows that his Word will give us meaning and purpose in life.

People of faith do not suddenly become that. The Christian grieves deeply over his loss and goes through the grief process. Eventually he understands that everything has not been taken from him and he wants to live again.

Hope and reality are based on faith in God's Word. Though we continue to struggle, we do find a new normal life. The struggle is hard if we try to do it on our own. All we need to do is relax and take God at his word, regardless of how we feel.

We may sometimes ask, "How do we put these ideas into practice in my life?"

First of all, we admit it. In other words, we acknowledge what has happened. We say it out loud (fill in the blanks), "I have lost _____." "_____ has died." "_____ has happened." After we have admitted honestly what has happened, we take the next step.

Next, vent it. We need to get the emotional stress out of our system, to tell someone exactly how we feel about the situation and loss. We must verbalize our anger and our sense of loss.

Next, release it. We must let go of our harmful feelings. If the dead are not permitted to die, then the living will not live.

We must express our grief when we lose a significant loved one, and we must go on living. Perhaps this is best expressed by the saying, "The eyes of the dead must be gently closed and the eyes of the living must be gently opened."

FIFTEEN
CARING AND
SELF-HELP GROUPS

Americans place great value on appearing to be strong, even when it means repressing feelings. This attitude is most unfortunate when people have to deal with the deep feelings that result from the loss of a close friend or loved one. People who live through the experience of seeing someone go through the process of dying usually develop strong empathy and gain helpful insights they didn't have before the experience. After they have gone through it, they understand the value of supporting friends who themselves have undergone the feelings.

Self-help groups have been formed to provide just this kind of system of emotional support to people in crisis. These groups may serve as learning resources, by providing knowledge about particular health problems. Some support groups may even become a sort of second family to people going through traumatic emotional problems. The goal for these groups, formed to aid those facing the death of friends and family members, is to help them reflect upon their own feelings and attitudes related to the process of death and dying.

Many groups across the nation have been formed that serve as models of caring and self-help for others; some can be adapted to the needs of any of our cities. Several of these groups are listed below:

THE CANDLELIGHTERS FOUNDATION
2025 Eye Street, N.W.
Suite 1011
Washington, DC 20006
202-659-5136

Candlelighters is an international, nonprofit organization of parents who have or have had children with cancer. This statement from their literature summarizes the organization's focus: "Candlelighters parents share the shock of diagnosis, the questions about treatment, the anxiety of waiting, the despair of relapse, the grief of death, the despondency of loss, the hope of remission, the joy of cure."

This group also makes available areas of help such as: newsletters, bibliographies, publications, speakers bureau, conferences, clearinghouse, and many other activities.

CARING
P. O. Box 1315
Abilene, TX 79604
915-698-4370

Caring is a distinctly Christian ministry and self-help group. The *Caring* team's commitments to each person whom they seek to serve are:

GOALS:
1. To assist those who are ill and their loved ones to find the strength from God for coping.
2. To identify with the emotional needs and practical

problems of those who are ill, sharing concrete suggestions that may be workable in the lives of those who are ill.

3. To openly declare the necessity of making a commitment to God as the foundation for any successful system of coping with illness.

4. To equip those who work with the ill with printed materials, tapes, and other resources so that their outreach may be meaningful and helpful.

PRINCIPLES:

Caring states several principles that guide their work with people:

1. We seek to understand the fears and uncertainties and unanswered questions that arise in the life of the patient and family, and to share helpful information and encouragement to meet this need.

2. We seek to tell people that they are not alone in fighting their serious illness, that some Christians care and are willing to provide various services to emotionally and spiritually support them in their battle.

3. We seek to encourage people to look to God in their time of crisis and to find in him the only permanent source of comfort, encouragement, and hope.

4. We believe that people are important; we seek to stay in touch with them as they are undergoing treatment so that we can lend encouragement in whatever way possible.

5. We try to empathize with those who live in an environment of pain and suffering and, while praying for them, to send them helpful tapes and printed materials that will be encouraging to them.

6. We utilize the personal experiences of [those] we know personally, to share possible solutions to the problems of depression, disappointment, aloneness, and other difficulties in the lives of patients and their families.

7. We try to supply nurses, doctors, ministers, and other interested individuals with tools that will help them deal personally with cancer patients in their own locale.

COMPASSIONATE FRIENDS

P. O. Box 1347
Oak Brook, IL 60521
312-323-5010

Compassionate Friends is a support group for bereaved parents who "need not walk alone. We are compassionate friends—people who care and share and listen to each other." The group discussions range from helping the grieving accept death to handling family holidays after the death of a child.

NATIONAL HOSPICE ORGANIZATION

1901 North Fort Myers Drive
Suite 401
Arlington, VA 22209
703-243-5900

PHILOSOPHY:
The hospice concept of self-help and group involvement can best be described as:
1. Ease the physical discomfort of the terminal patient by employing pharmaceutical and advanced clinical techniques for effective symptom control.
2. Ease the psychological discomfort of the terminal patient through programs allowing for active participation in scheduled activities or periods of peaceful withdrawal as determined by the patient.
3. Aid in maintaining the emotional equilibrium of the patient and the family as they go through the trau-

matic experience of progressive disease and ultimately the final separation of death.

PRIORITIES:

Hospice is a program that desires to meet a wide range of physical, psychological, social, and spiritual needs. This health-care program identifies ten of its priorities:

1. Service availability to home care patients and in-patients on a twenty-four-hour-a-day, seven-day-a-week, on-call basis with emphasis on availability of medical and nursing skills.

2. Home care service in collaboration with inpatient families.

3. Knowledge and expertise in control of symptoms (physical, psychological, social, and spiritual).

4. The provision of care by an interdisciplinary team.

5. Physician-directed services.

6. Central administration and coordination of services.

7. Use of volunteers as an integral part of the health-care team.

8. Acceptance of the program based on health needs, not ability to pay.

9. Treatment of the patient and family together as a unit of care.

10. A bereavement follow-up service.

NRT-AARP-AIM

1909 K Street, N.W.
Washington, DC 20049

The National Retired Teachers Association, the American Association of Retired Persons, and the Action for Independent Maturity (NRT-AARP-AIM) have together formed a caring organization. This combined group has formed a network for living through grief bereavement.

Their organization offers an outreach program that helps people on an individual as well as a group basis. Their main priorities are to provide:
1. Telephone service for referral information.
2. A public education program for family adjustment.
3. Counseling for financial and legal affairs.
4. Referral counseling.

SHARE AND CARE

North Memorial Medical Center
3220 Lowry Avenue North
Minneapolis, MN 55422

Share and Care have presented a model for the medical professionals. Representatives of physicians, nurses, social services, and chaplaincy staffs foster close relationships among terminally ill patients and family members. They minister to one another by getting involved in one another's problems during weekly meetings.

Spouses and other family members often continue to come to meetings even after the patient dies. Through continued contact with the support group, survivors share their grief experiences and help others who may be facing similar problems or situations.

MAKE TODAY COUNT

P. O. Box 303
Burlington, IA 52601

Make Today Count is an international mutual support organization made up of local chapters. These groups bring together those persons who are affected by serious illness so that they help each other learn to live life in a positive and meaningful manner. In the words of the organization's founder, Orville Kelly, "I do not look upon each day as another day closer to death, but as another day of life, to be appreciated and enjoyed."

Make Today Count is dedicated to improving the quality of life of those who have been touched by serious illness. Meetings are open to those who have had life-threatening diseases. Their families and friends are also welcomed as well as interested professionals and other community members.

The goals of this self-help group are:

1. To help the patient and his or her family cope with life-threatening illnesses.

2. To improve the quality of life for all persons with serious illness.

3. To identify emotional problems of life-threatening illnesses and teach people to cope with them.

4. To promote openness and honesty in discussing and dealing with a serious illness.

5. To assist the professional in communicating and meeting the needs of the patient, family, and friends who are faced with a life-threatening problem.

THE SELF-HELP CENTER
1600 Dodge Avenue
Suite S-122
Evanston, IL 60204
312-218-0470

This center serves as a clearinghouse for self-help and mutual help groups. Groups have now been organized for sufferers of all the seventeen disease categories recognized by the World Health Organization. This center is particularly helpful in locating the appropriate group nearest you.

AMEND
4324 Berrywick Terrace
St. Louis, MO 63128
314-487-7582

AMEND stands for Aiding a Mother Experiencing Neonatal Death. This group began as an offshoot from Lifeseekers, a voluntary organization that provides life-saving equipment to hospitals. The primary goal of this group is to offer support by phone or personal visit to mothers who have lost a baby before birth or at the time of birth. They have trained lay counselors who have experienced the loss of a child.

THE NATIONAL SIDS FOUNDATION
2 Metro Plaza
Suite 205
8420 Professional Place
Landover, MD 20785

SIDS stands for Sudden Infant Death Syndrome. This national office supports local community chapters for parents who have lost children to SIDS or SIDS-related symptoms. They provide films, training support materials, and parent-to-parent referral services.

THE SAMARITANS
500 Commonwealth Avenue
Boston, MA 02215
617-536-2460
617-247-0220 (for emergencies only)

The Samaritans are a special group of volunteers trained to respond to individuals who are considering suicide. They also provide counsel to people who have lost a relative or friend to suicide. The emergency telephone service is covered twenty-four hours a day.

SHARE

St. John's Hospital
800 East Carpenter
Springfield, IL 62769
217-544-6464

This group has more than eighty chapters in thirty states. They focus on the needs of parents who have lost a baby due to miscarriage, stillbirth, or early infant death. Most of the volunteers are bereaved parents. They are hospital staff members as well as lay workers. This group offers educational and organizational materials.

THEOS FOUNDATION

Office Building-Penn Hills Mall
Suite 410
Pittsburgh, PA 15235
412-243-4299

THEOS stands for They Help Each Other Spiritually. It is a group that offers self-help assistance to young and middle-aged widows. They have a monthly magazine and several brochures. Self-help materials are available from this group.

PARENTS WITHOUT PARTNERS

7910 Woodmont Avenue
Suite 1008
Bethesda, MD 20814
301-654-8850

Parents Without Partners is a nonsectarian organization which has more than seven hundred chapters. The members of this organization are concerned with the welfare of single parents and their children. Their motto is "Sharing by Caring."

CONCLUSION

Each person who has read this book has probably identified with some dimension of death and dying that has been presented. Each person has looked at the subject from a different set of eyes or personal perspective. The book has been written in general terms so that it could be understood by a wide range of persons that have come or will come in contact with the process of death and dying.

My goal has been to help people reflect upon their own feelings and attitudes related to dying, death, and grief. Perhaps the reflective thinking has helped to open the door on a taboo subject and the book will become an aid to helping people to help themselves.

More than three hundred years ago a philosopher named La Rochefoucauld-Liancourt said that "the human mind is as little capable to contemplate death for any long length of time as the eye is able to look at the sun." It is normal to advance and retreat in our viewing of the aspects of death. Yet, the need to face the subject remains as important as ever if we are to be prepared for that time.

As I finished writing, I have disclosed how little I

know about the mystery of death. In many ways, I am ashamed of how little I know about death and dying. Yet never have I enjoyed life more than when I started having the courage to begin facing death and living life.

NOTES

CHAPTER 1

[1]Ideas adapted and used by permission. "Patient's Bill of Rights." *Nursing Outlook*. 24:29, 1979.

[2]Ideas adapted and used by permission. Make Today Count, San Diego Chapter, P. O. Box 15203, San Diego, CA 92115.

[3]Department of Health and Human Services, Human Resources Code, chapter 102.

CHAPTER 2

[1]"The Dying Person's Bill of Rights." Southwestern Michigan Inservice Education Council, Wayne State University, Detroit, Mich.

CHAPTER 3

[1]Ideas adapted and used by permission. Make Today Count, Box 222, Osage Beach, MO 65065.

[2]The Christian Affirmation of Life. This statement was developed by the Catholic Hospital Association of the United States.

[3]Ideas adapted and used by permission. Mary Myer, "Dealing with Death," *America*, September 3, 1977.

CHAPTER 5

[1]Ideas adapted and used by permission. Larry Richards and Paul Johnson, *Death and the Caring Community* (Portland, Oreg.: Multnomah Press, 1980), 61.

CHAPTER 6

[1]For an in-depth treatment, see Jim Towns, *Growing Through Grief* (Anderson, Ind.: Warner Press, 1984).

CHAPTER 7

[1]Ideas adapted and used by permission. Anya Foos-Graber, *Deathing* (Reading, Mass.: Addison-Wesley, 1984).

[2]*Mosby's Medical and Nursing Dictionary*, 2nd edition (St. Louis: C. V. Mosby Company, 1986), 223.

[3]Billy Graham, *Angels* (New York: Pocket Books, 1976).

CHAPTER 8

[1]Ideas used by permission. Elizabeth Kubler-Ross, *On Death and Dying* (New York: Macmillan Publishing Company, 1969).

CHAPTER 9
[1]"Ad hoc Committee of the Harvard School to Examine the Definition of Brain Death," *Journal of the American Medical Assocation*, 205 (1968), 337-340.

CHAPTER 10
[1]Ideas paraphrased and used by permission. Larry Richards and Paul Johnson, M.D., *Death and the Caring Community* (Portland, Oreg.: Multnomah Press, 1980).

CHAPTER 11
[1]Ideas adapted and used by permission. Mc. C. McCoy, *To Die with Style* (Nashville: Abingdon, 1974).

CHAPTER 12
[1]Used by permission. News America Syndicate and Minneapolis *Tribune*.

CHAPTER 13
[1]Used by permission. Code of Professional Practices for Funeral Directors (originally adopted Nov. 1965; revised in 1969 and 1972), National Funeral Directors Association.

[2]Ideas used by permission. National Selected Morticians.

CHAPTER 14
[1]For an in-depth treatment, see Jim Towns, *Growing Through Grief* (Anderson, Ind.: Warner Press, 1984).

SELECTED
BIBLIOGRAPHY

Anderson, J. Kerby. *Life, Death and Beyond*. Grand Rapids: Zondervan, 1980.

Annas, George J. *The Rights of Hospital Patients*. New York: Avon, 1975.

Billheimer, Paul. *Destined to Overcome*. Minneapolis: Bethany House, 1982.

————. *Don't Waste Your Sorrows*. Fort Washington, Penn.: Christian Literature Crusade, 1977.

Cousins, Norman. *Anatomy of an Illness*. New York: W. W. Norton, 1979.

Frankl, Viktor. *Man's Search for Meaning*. New York: Pocket Books, Simon & Schuster, 1980.

Graham, Billy. *Angels*. New York: Doubleday, 1975.

Grollman, Earl A. *Talking about Death*. Boston: Beacon Press, 1970.

Grubb, Norman. *The Law of Faith*. Fort Washington, Penn.: Christian Literature Crusade, 1977.

————. *The Liberating Secret*. Fort Washington, Penn.: Christian Literature Crusade, 1955.

Hamilton, Michael P., and Helen F. Reed, eds. *A Hospice Handbook*. Grand Rapids: Eerdmans, 1980.

Jackson, Edgar N. *The Many Faces of Grief*. Center City, Minn.: Hazelden, 1977.

————. *Understanding Grief*. Nashville: Abingdon Press, 1957.

Jourard, Sidney. *The Transparent Self*. New York: Van Nostrand Reinhold Co., 1971.

Kelly, Orville. *Make Today Count*. New York: Delacorte, 1975.

————. *Until Tomorrow Comes*. New York: Everest House, 1979.

Kopp, Ruth, and Stephen Sorensen. *Terminal Illness*. Grand Rapids: Zondervan, 1980.

Kubler-Ross, Elizabeth. *On Death and Dying*. New York: Macmillan, 1974.

Lewis, C. S. *A Grief Observed*. New York: Seabury Press, 1961.

————. *The Problem of Pain*. New York: Macmillan, 1962.

Long, James W. *The Essential Guide to Prescription Drugs*. New York: Harper & Row, 1982.

Lovett, C. S. *Death: Graduation to Glory*. Baldwin Park, Calif.: Personal Christianity, 1974.

Mayeroff, Milton. *On Caring*. New York: Harper & Row, 1972.

Minirth, Frank B., and Paul D. Meier. *Happiness Is a Choice*. Grand Rapids: Baker Book House, 1978.

————. *Counseling and the Nature of Man*. Grand Rapids: Baker Book House, 1982.

Moody, Raymond A., Jr. *Life after Life*. New York: Bantam Books, 1977.

————. *Reflections on Life after Life*. New York: Bantam Books, 1978.

Murphree, Jon T. *A Loving God and a Suffering World*. Downers Grove, Ill.: Intervarsity Press, 1981.

Nee, Watchman. *The Normal Christian Life*. Wheaton, Ill.: Tyndale House Publishers, 1977.

Peck, M. Scott. *The Road Less Traveled*. New York: Simon & Schuster, 1978.

Phillips, J. B. *Your God Is Too Small*. New York: Macmillan Co., 1963.

Rawlings, Maurice. *Beyond Death's Door*. New York: Bantam, 1979.

Robertson, Pat, and Bob Slosser. *The Secret Kingdom*. Nashville: Thomas Nelson, 1982.

Schaeffer, Edith. *Affliction*. Old Tappan, N.J.: Fleming Revell, 1978.

Schuller, Robert. *The Be Happy Attitudes*. Waco, Tex.: Word, 1985.

Sullender, R. Scott. *Grief and Growth*. New York: Paulist Press, 1985.

Tengbom, Mildred. *Why Waste Your Illness?* Minneapolis: Augsburg, 1984.

Towns, Jim. *Faith Stronger Than Death*. Anderson, Ind.: Warner Press, 1975.

———. *Growing Through Grief*. Anderson, Ind.: Warner Press, 1984.

———. *Singles Alive!* Gretna, La.: Pelican Publishing, 1984.

———. *Solo Flight*. Wheaton, Ill.: Tyndale House Publishers, 1980.

Whitaker, Donald. *The Divine Connection: Feel Better and Live Longer*. Shreveport: Huntington House, 1983.

Ziglar, Zig. *See You at the Top*. Gretna, La.: Pelican Publishing, 1977.